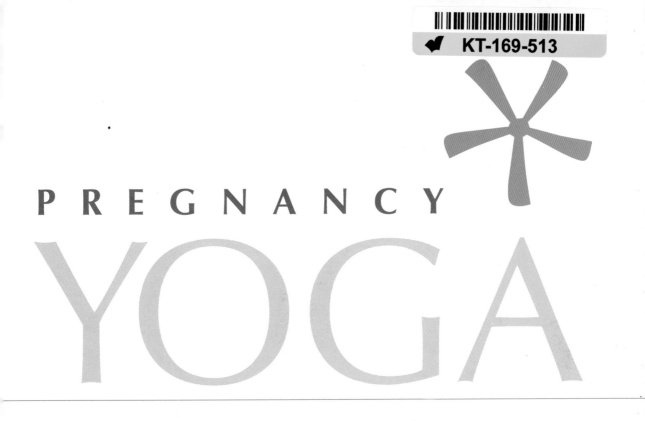

PREGNANCY
YOGA

ENERGISING, INVIGORATING, STRENGTHENING

SAMANTHA MAGEE

CONTENTS

FOREWORD

Being pregnant and giving birth are among the most natural things in the world – a time when a woman's body is at its full potential. However, many women can find this time unsettling due to increased hormone levels and the variety of physical changes taking place on top of the pressures of everyday life. The increase in medical intervention in Western society has made pregnancy and childbirth a lot safer. But as a result the whole process can seem very clinical and complex at times, which means that some women can feel detached from the natural experience. This is a shame as every woman deserves to feel fully connected with her own body and her unborn baby at this special time.

Yoga can be an invaluable tool in making pregnancy and birth all-round easier and more positive experiences. Highly recommended by birthing experts and medical practitioners, yoga is an ancient Indian practice that combines physical postures with breathing, meditation and visualisation techniques in order to maintain balance in both the body and mind. Postures (*asanas*) provide a gentle form of stretching and

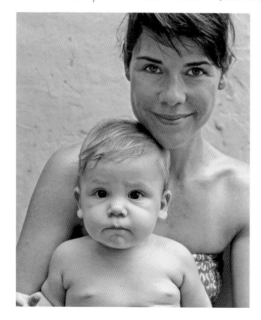

strengthening that keeps the body fit and supple during pregnancy, while breathing (pranayama), meditation and visualisation techniques help expectant mothers to accept change, maintain a positive mental outlook and deepen the mind-body connection with their unborn baby.

The practice of yoga also acts as a maintenance programme on a basic level to support all the major systems, keeping the skeletal, muscular, respiratory, cardiovascular, nervous, endocrine and reproductive systems in balance as much as possible throughout your pregnancy. A regular practice can also help to minimise common pregnancy symptoms, such as morning sickness and constipation, ease labour and help to restore your body after childbirth.

The experience of my first pregnancy was a wonderful one for me but also a bit of a shock. Having practised yoga for many years and maintained a high level of health and fitness, I was used to feeling stable and balanced. Then, overnight, I suddenly had to deal with a torrent of increased hormones and rapidly changing emotions as well as the vast changes that were happening to my body and my life.

Throughout my pregnancy, yoga helped me to maintain a sense of balance and perspective. It allowed me to remain physically strong and vital, but, more importantly, my regular practice gave me mental and emotional stability when change was all around. Having to accept that I could no longer do my favourite stronger yoga poses, such as Floor Bow or Crane, helped me to expand my concept of yoga and to enjoy a more deeply centred practice. Through having a greater understanding of my body's capacity and embracing my natural instincts and intuition, I feel I connected deeply with my unborn child and gave him a strong foundation for the future.

When I first needed to adapt my practice to my own pregnancy, I found a scarcity of information on the subject. So I have written this book to support future practitioners, and I hope that this guide will help you, too, to enjoy and embrace your experience of pregnancy more profoundly. The choice of postures and clear, step-by-step guidelines for each one make the programmes easily accessible for beginners, while information on how to adapt an existing yoga practice to one that is suitable for pregnancy means that the book is also ideal for more experienced practitioners.

My hope is that this book will empower pregnant women to practise regularly, become more connected with their natural power, remain strong and healthy, and deliver beautiful, balanced, strong and confident children.

Samantha Magee

PREPARING FOR PRACTICE

For some of you, this may be the first time you have done yoga, so it's important that you have some background information on how to prepare for practice in order to get the most from it. And for those of you who practise regularly, it's always good to go back to the basics to make sure you haven't slipped into any bad habits.

When practising yoga, choose times that suit you and that can fit in regularly with your schedule – and mark these into your diary. That way, doing yoga will be easier and more enjoyable for you. Ideally you should strive for a consistent practice at pre-decided times each week. The more your body gets programmed through the exercises and techniques, the more positively it will respond.

Choose a private space that is clean, clear of furniture, well ventilated and at a good temperature so you don't feel too hot or cold. Avoid high heat and humidity. Ensure that your chosen space has adequate lighting and try to make sure that it offers a sturdy wall for support as well as enough space for a yoga mat and any props you want to use (see p. 28).

Before you begin a yoga session, turn off your phone and let friends and family know not to bother you during your yoga time. If you like music, play something that suits your mood – whether inspirational and uplifting, or calm and restorative. But always allow yourself a few minutes of silence at the end of a session where you can connect fully with your mind.

Wear loose, comfortable clothing that allows easy movement. Supportive tops or vests will help to keep your beautifully expanding bust in check.

Remove all jewellery, glasses and watches. Also remove socks so that your feet can grip well onto your yoga mat to maintain solid footing.

Make sure to stay well hydrated both before and during any exercise. It is best to practise on an empty stomach, but you might benefit from eating something light and easily digestible half an hour to an hour beforehand to keep blood sugar levels up or to stave off nausea. If so, suggestions are a banana, a handful of dried fruit, a slice of toast, and/or a cup of warm water or herbal tea.

You should also support your yoga practice with a healthy diet in your day-to-day life: the healthier you become through a combination of a well-rounded diet and regular exercise, the more connected you will feel to your practice and the more joy you will gain from it.

Before you begin any of the yoga techniques, first familiarise yourself in full with all the safety aspects (see p. 11), as well as the step-by-step guidance for each posture, or sequence.

Once you are ready to start, do so slowly and carefully, referring to the book as often as you need to. As you become more confident, you can practise more intuitively.

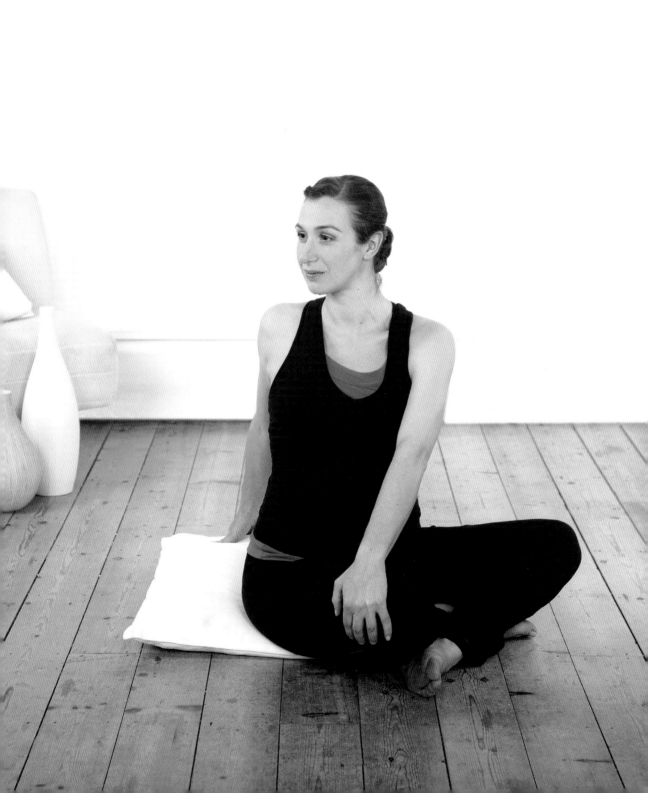

THE IMPORTANCE OF ALIGNMENT

Yoga is one of the best forms of exercise to undertake when pregnant because it emphasises gentle stretches, strengthening and opening while maintaining awareness of alignment and proper technique. Proper physical alignment is always key to a safe and effective yoga practice. But it is all the more crucial during pregnancy, as your skeletal system is under such pressure as a result of your increasing weight, your opening joints (due to the effect of the hormone relaxin – see p. 11) and your baby's position. Proper alignment will help to support your weight-bearing joints as you go about your daily business, as well as providing a strong foundation for your yoga practice. So it is important to avoid forming bad habits in your posture and alignment. There are a series of simple rules and checks to remember before you begin standing or seated postures to ensure correct alignment for the forthcoming pose.

Simple rules for standing

- Keep your feet hip-width apart and parallel to create a stable base. When your feet are correctly aligned, the rest of your body will naturally follow.
- Distribute your weight equally over the front, back and sides of your feet.
- Avoid locking your knees so that no unnecessary pressure is placed on your joints.
- Make sure you neither slouch nor overarch your back – when standing, try pulling up through the top of your head to maintain the natural curvature in your spine (this curvature will increase during pregnancy).
- Keep your chin level – neither too tucked in nor too raised up.

Simple rules for sitting

- Position the base of your spine against the back of a chair.
- Place your legs hip-width apart and your feet flat on the floor. Alternatively, place books or yoga blocks under your feet if they do not naturally sit flat due to the height of the chair.
- Tilt your pelvis slightly forwards and lengthen up through your spine, keeping your head centred over your spinal column.
- Rest your hands gently on your thighs, keeping your shoulders back and down to promote free, easy breathing.

YOGA SAFETY

Safety – for both yourself and your unborn child – is the top priority when doing any exercise while pregnant, so take time to read this section a few times before hitting the mat, especially if you are new to yoga. And always check with a medical professional before starting a new exercise programme.

- Yoga can be practised every day if you feel like it but it's important not to overdo it. Aim for a regular practice, rather than an intermittent one.
- Try starting with 15–20 minutes minimum at least twice a week and building up.
- Avoid practising in high heat and humidity.
- Practise bare-foot so that your feet can grip onto the mat to maintain solid footing.
- Never do too rigorous a practice while pregnant. However, if you are already active and physically fit, the poses can be performed to about 70 per cent of your pre-pregnancy level, taking on board modifications relevant to your changing body and being sure to rest if you get tired.
- Maintain a focus on breathing naturally throughout your practice in order to connect your mind and body. This will result in increased awareness and intuition.
- Ensure that you can always breathe easily – enough to still carry on a conversation.
- Be careful not to overstretch as levels of the hormone relaxin increase during pregnancy to loosen your ligaments in preparation for child birth. Since ligaments and tendons do not have the same elasticity as muscle, it may be hard for them to regain their shape once the relaxin leaves your body.

- Avoid strong jarring movements that will place additional strain on joints during this period of increased flexibility.
- Always maintain a stable foundation going into, during and coming out of poses.
- Use props such as chairs, walls and blocks (see p. 28) if you feel they will be helpful for extra support.
- Take a common sense approach to your practice and be your own best yoga teacher. This involves being aware of, and adapting to, whatever your current needs are – both physical and emotional.
- Remember to trust yourself fully. If something does not feel right, then don't do it or try to take some of the effort out of the position so it feels more comfortable.
- Stay positive and open-minded. At times you might not feel like engaging fully in your yoga session, but the positive effects will be worth it in the end.
- If energy is low, place your focus on gentle postures, and more breathing and relaxation.
- Refer back to the step-by-step guidance in this book periodically to make sure you are doing the postures correctly.

HOW TO USE THIS BOOK

By following these guidelines you will benefit from a full yoga class that includes stretching, strengthening, bending, twisting, balancing and, of course, resting. Here's to a happy, healthy pregnancy.

Read this introductory section thoroughly for background and safety information before practising the postures in the book, whether you are new to yoga or an experienced practitioner. You'll also find a section covering some of the fundamentals of pregnancy yoga (see pp. 14–31), guiding your through the stages of your pregnancy, your nutritional needs, adapting your practice, optional props, and any other information relevant to the practice of yoga during pregnancy.

The exercise section of the book then opens with the warm-up sequence, which is suitable throughout your pregnancy. Do several rounds of the Sun Salutation sequence (see pp. 34–39) either as a yoga session in its own right or as a warm-up before doing the relevant trimester sequence.

The subsequent chapters are divided into postures and modifications best suited for your body during the first (see pp. 44–61), second (see pp. 62–83) and third (see pp. 84–99) trimesters. Always be sure to choose the posture variations

that feel most relevant to you at the time. During any yoga session, rest in Child's pose (see p. 122) any time you feel tired.

After the birth of your baby, when your body needs time to recover, practise only the postnatal sequence (see p. 100–119), which incorporates a warm-up of its own.

Whatever stage of your pregnancy, finish your yoga session with the relaxation exercises (see pp. 120–129), which can also be practised on their own any time you need to unwind.

In addition to and as part of your physical yoga routines, do your preferred selection of breathing and meditation techniques (see pp. 130–139) any time you feel the need for increased calm, clarity or energy balancing. These are helpful in learning to deal with the emotional rollercoaster that many women experience during their pregnancy.

After 12 to 16 weeks you may feel strong enough to resume elements of your prenatal or regular practice.

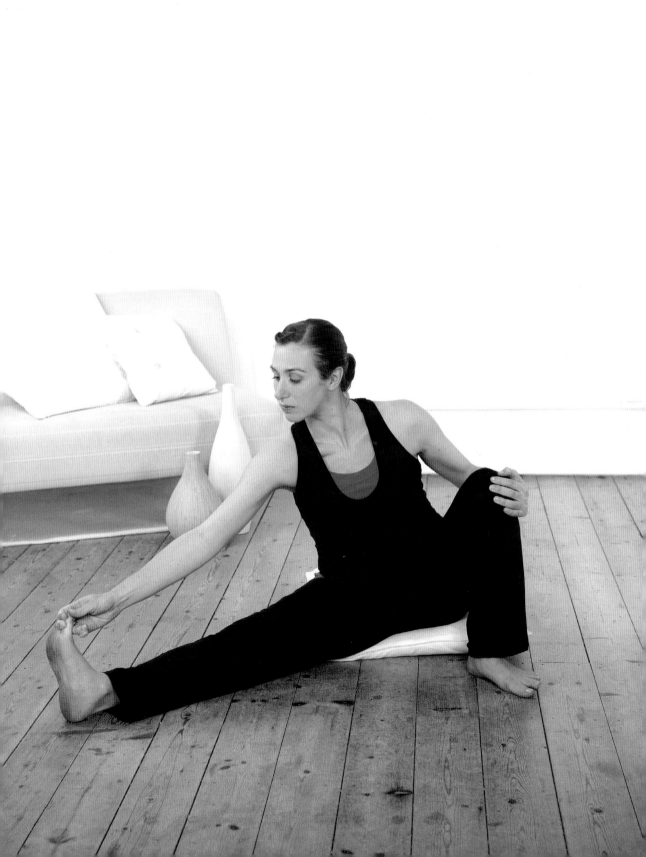

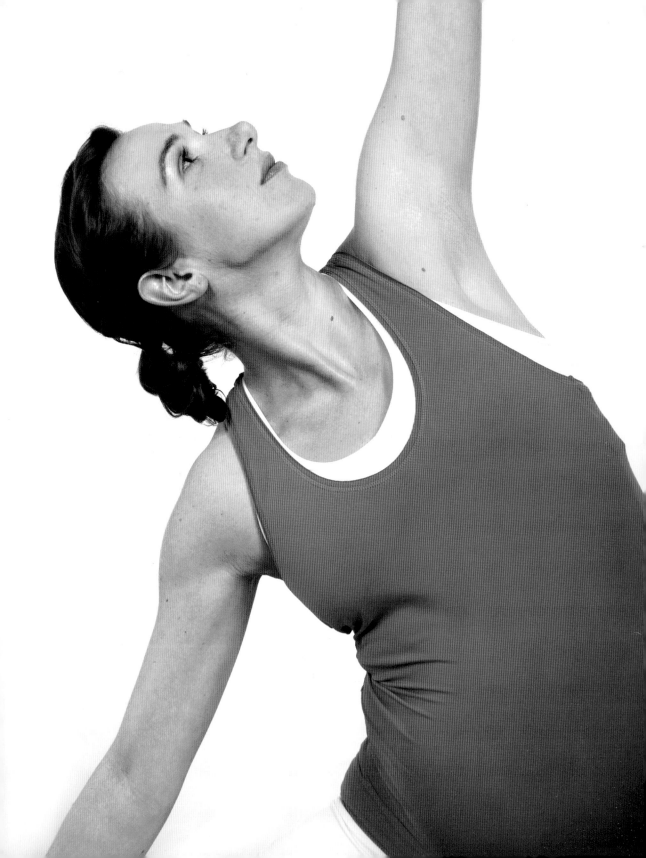

THE FUNDAMENTALS
OF PREGNANCY YOGA

Whether you have picked up this book to gain a few simple tips to make your pregnancy easier or are a regular yoga practitioner looking to adapt your practice for pregnancy, the pages that follow will provide guidance on how to tap into a holistic yoga system that can nurture and support you not only during pregnancy and labour but also following the birth of your baby. This chapter provides invaluable information on what to expect both physically and emotionally during each trimester of pregnancy, as well as once your baby is born; how, broadly speaking, to adapt your yoga to suit each trimester; the fundamental dietary requirements at each stage; and advice on different props to use.

With first-hand experience of how powerful a yoga practice can be, women often continue practising after birth to help them to get their body back in shape as well as to support them with the emotional changes of new motherhood. And many even introduce their children to yoga.

STAGES OF PREGNANCY

Pregnancy is defined by three distinct trimesters, the details of which are outlined in the pages that follow. Each period lasts approximately three months, with the mother's body adapting to support the growing foetus in preparation for the baby's birth.

It is important to have an understanding of these three stages as each one involves different developmental factors for both the mother and baby, which need to be taken into account when practising yoga. There is, of course, also the labour itself and the postnatal (afterbirth) period, which have their own sets of requirements.

The first trimester

The first trimester starts at the time of conception and continues with the development of the embryo, which officially becomes a foetus in the second month. By the end of the first trimester, the foetus is starting to show teeth, can swallow, has fully developed hands, and its gender is usually established. A healthy baby tends to be approximately 7.6 to 10cm (3 to 4in) in length and weigh around 28g (1oz) at this point.

During this trimester, the mother is likely to experience symptoms such as tender breasts, nausea and vomiting due to morning sickness, slight tightness in the abdomen and strong energetic shifts as a great deal of energy is being devoted to the creation of the child. Emotionally, the first trimester can be volatile as it is such an intense period of transition, with a large increase in hormone levels.

It is during this period of substantial foetal development that there is the highest risk of miscarriage, as the placenta is not yet fully formed to support the baby and the hormones are unsteady, so this should be a time of gentle movement, energy maintenance and utmost safety.

Whether you are a new or regular yoga practitioner, the first trimester is a time to:

- Go slow – rest, when it feels right, in postures such as Child's pose (see p. 122), Legs up the Wall (see p. 124) or Corpse pose (see p. 128) to maintain energy levels.
- Practise breathing exercises, starting with Full Yogic Breathing (see p. 26).
- Develop pelvic awareness through postures such as Hip Rolls (see p. 48), Bridge (see p. 56), Cat (see p. 52) and Cowface (see p. 54).
- Stimulate circulation to the pelvis and lower extremities with hip-opening postures, such as Arm and Leg Extension (see p. 76) and Gentle Lunge (see p. 41), as well as Butterfly (see p. 46), Hip Rolls (see p. 48) and Happy Baby (see p. 60).
- Focus on positive physical alignment to create a strong foundation for the body as it undergoes all the change – Mountain pose is ideal for this (see p. 34).

The second trimester

The second trimester lasts from the beginning of the fourth to the beginning of the seventh month of pregnancy. This period is marked by the placenta being fully functional and hormone levels beginning to stabilise. The uterus is enlarging with the growth of the foetus, so the baby bump will be starting to show. As a result there can be pressure on the belly from the expanding muscles and ligaments of the pelvis.

Yoga advice for the first trimester

- Aim to maintain a gentle flow going in and out of each pose.
- Minimise any jolting actions that can stress the body; this includes eliminating jumping into poses if you are a regular practitioner.
- Remain highly aware of how your body feels as you perform all movements and slowly come out of any posture in which you experience discomfort.
- Any twisting poses should focus on the upper back so that there is no strong compression to the abdomen. The twisting postures in this book have been chosen to reflect this.
- The foetus is still small and protected by the pelvis, so lying on the stomach is fine if it feels alright.

Blood supply is increasing to accommodate for the baby, and hormones such as relaxin, which loosens your ligaments in preparation for child birth, are in more abundance, so mothers can experience swollen gums, changes in circulation and body heat, as well as less stability in the joints. Mothers can also notice changes to complexion and hair due to hormonal shifts, and may also experience heartburn, constipation and nasal congestion. The main thing to remember is that these symptoms will all be short-lived.

As the baby needs more energy to grow, your appetite is likely to increase, so it becomes even more important to focus on proper diet and nutrition (see pp. 22–23).

Through the second trimester your baby's finger and toe prints form and the eyes open. By the fifth month, your baby can hear your voice so this is an ideal time to talk, sing and play music to your bump to increase your bond. Don't be surprised to get a strong response to this added stimulation, especially by the sixth month, when your baby will be moving about more and might even suck its thumb, yawn and stretch. By this stage, the baby will also be able to distinguish between light and dark, and teeth and bones will be denser.

The best thing about the second trimester is the return of your natural energy, so this is a time to:

- Work on building strength and stamina – practising several rounds of the Sun Salutation sequence (see pp. 34–39) any time you want is great for this but remember to rest if needed.
- Build upper and lower body strength through Warrior positions (see pp. 64–67), Wide-leg

Squats (see p. 72), Gentle Plank (see p. 78) and Easy Push-ups (see p. 79).

- Continue to open and support the pelvic muscles with hip-openers, such as Bridge (see p. 56) and Hip Rolls (see p. 48).
- Begin deeper relaxation and meditation practices, such as Blowing a Feather Breath (see p. 134) and Abundance meditation (see p. 134), to increase the mother-baby connection.

All this work will support and sustain you during labour and after birth when energy can be low.

The third trimester

By the third trimester all your baby's systems are fully functioning: nails are getting longer, hair thicker, and body weight and fat stores are increasing so that the baby can provide its own energy upon arrival into the wider world. As a result of this growth, there is less room inside you for the baby to move, which can put strain on your pelvis and back. By full term, your baby will, on average, be 51cm (20in) in length and weigh around 3.4kg (7.5lb).

Common symptoms for the mother during this period are an increased level of fatigue, backache, heartburn and breathlessness. As the hormone relaxin is at its highest level, added strain can be felt in the joints, so now is a time to focus on remaining rested and comfortable without overdoing it. It is therefore good to:

- Really bring your attention to correct alignment (see p. 10) in order to support the major joints.

Yoga advice for the second trimester

- Your baby is increasing in size, and your internal organs are being shifted to accommodate for this, so avoid intense abdominal work such as classic sit-ups or crunches.
- Do, however, maintain gentle stomach strengthening exercises such as Cat (see p. 52) and Gentle Plank (see p. 78) to condition your belly and help it return to original strength after birth.
- Be aware of any numbness when lying on your back due to pressure on major arteries. If you feel this, limit your time in this position or shift to a side-lying position.
- Gentle inversions such as Downward Dog (see p. 36) are fine if they feel ok but it's best to avoid full inversions such as Shoulderstand and Headstand from here on in.

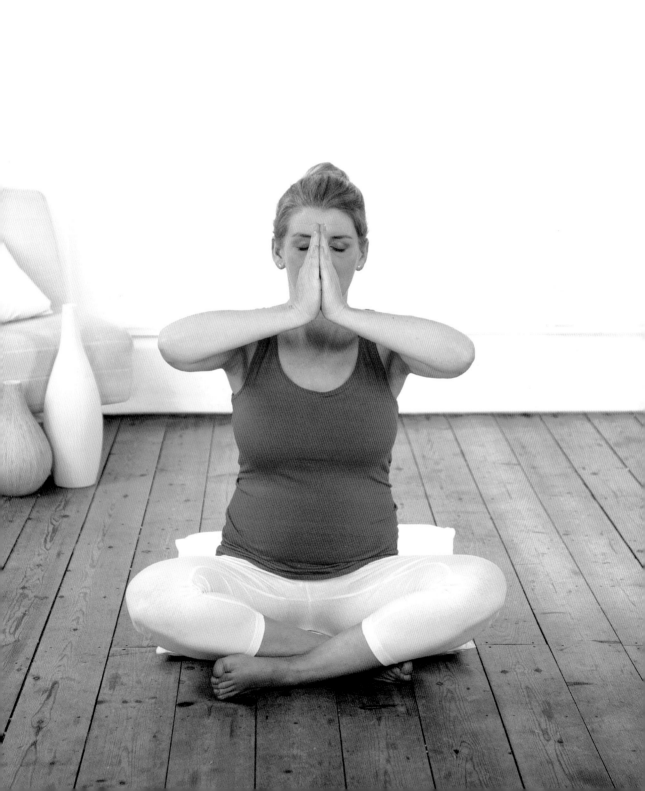

- Start using more props to support your body in postures (see p. 28).
- Perform relaxation poses (see pp. 120–129) with cushions and blankets so that your body can fully unwind.
- Limit the time you spend lying on your back.
- Continue to practise breathing and meditation techniques (see pp. 130–139) to help to foster patience and a sense of calm as you approach your due date.

Labour

Now comes the big day you've been patiently waiting for! Labour is generally divided into three stages:

- onset of contractions
- full labour, or pushing the baby out
- delivery of the placenta

These stages will vary in duration for each mother but birthing a baby is likely to be the most physically demanding experience that a woman ever goes through.

   Contractions will be intense and labour hard work but all your mind and body preparation during pregnancy will now prove worthwhile. Your physical yoga practice will have developed within you the necessary strength and stamina to sustain the energy required for labour, while breathing exercises, meditations and visualisations will help to keep your mind focused and calm. As a result, your body can remain as relaxed as possible, and delivery of your beautiful new baby will hopefully be smooth and safe.

Yoga advice for the third trimester

- Continue practising the Sun Salutation sequence (see pp. 34–39) if it feels comfortable but, if needed, modify the Downward Dog (see p. 36) to a kneeling variation, especially after the baby has moved into the birth position.
- Practise Deep Squat in Prayer (see p. 88), Hip Rolls (see pp. 48–49), Wide-leg Seated Stretches (see pp. 94–97) and Seated Spinal Twists (see pp. 98–99) to support the growing impact on your body.
- Really focus on breathing deeply during your practice in order to calm the mind, especially if you start to feel overwhelmed by the thought of impending labour and motherhood.
- Consider doing exercises such as Welcoming the Baby meditation (see p. 138) or Birthing Visualisation (see p. 136) in squat positions to encourage the baby to move into the correct position for labour.
- Limit time in inverted positions such as Downward Dog.

Postnatal period

Your baby has arrived and you are now officially a mother – congratulations! The postnatal period is a rollercoaster ride with the first days after birth filled with euphoria, excitement and adrenaline as you get used to your new baby and the routine of feeding, burping, changing and rocking.

Depending on the type of labour you experienced, whether a natural birth or caesarean section, it is very important that you rest and fully heal from the birth experience. During the first six weeks post-birth, take every opportunity to nap while your baby is sleeping, accept help from others and eat nutritious food to support yourself and to build healthy milk production for your baby. Remember that you have this child for the rest of its life, so you will need precious energy to support it as the months progress.

Your body has changed dramatically through nine months of pregnancy and labour, so physically your body needs time to re-align and strengthen, and for your organs, joints and ligaments to return to normal. Emotionally, hormones are still racing through your body, so you can feel elated one minute and down the next. Yoga postures and breathing will help to stabilise your emotions and support your body, which can help to prevent the onset of postnatal depression. This is the time to:

- Begin practising gentle yoga postures when you feel ready or after a six-week medical clearance if you had a C-section.
- Building stamina and muscular strength will take time, so practise yoga little and often.

- Focus on the proper alignment of your spine when standing, kneeling, sitting or lying down.
- Rest often during and after yoga routines.
- Remember to practise breathing deeply through your nose throughout your yoga session and you can resume breath retention practices.
- Lying on your back feels great after birth, so place your baby on your chest and do gentle stretches and twists.
- After six weeks, you can begin to exercise more fully, but remember that your body is not the same as before pregnancy. So practise caution especially when focusing on the pelvic, abdominal and back muscles.
- Follow each yoga practice with relaxation postures, which can be performed holding your baby. This is a great way to recharge and bond.

NUTRITIONAL NEEDS

For many women becoming pregnant for the first time means becoming more acutely aware of the importance of proper nutrition as you are now thinking about the health and well-being of your unborn baby as well as yourself.

By eating moderate amounts of wholesome food during pregnancy, you and your baby will obtain all the necessary nutrients to grow strong and healthy. Resisting the all-too-common temptation to 'eat for two' will allow your weight gain to remain reflective of what both you and your baby need in terms of energy (a pregnant woman only needs approximately 100 to 300 additional calories a day).

This sensible approach will not only mean you can stay light on your feet throughout your pregnancy but will also increase your chances of returning more quickly to your natural body weight after the birth.

The somewhat restricted diet during pregnancy – no alcohol, no soft cheeses, reducing caffeine, avoiding certain shellfish such as oysters, and potentially not wanting to eat certain foods due to morning sickness – can feel difficult to adjust to on top of all the other physical changes. But try to embrace the chance to form healthy eating habits that will carry forward to the well-being of your entire family.

A regular yoga practice will help you to become more intuitive about your body's physical needs, so try to tune into this when it comes to food, too. Having a few treats here and there is fine, but you and your baby need good all-round nutritional fitness to develop happily and healthily.

In the first trimester
With hormone swings and morning sickness, try to eat little and often in order to maintain balanced blood sugar and energy levels. Drinking ginger tea works well for calming nausea.

In the second trimester
Appetite will increase and nausea will subside, so enjoy eating a wide a variety of whole, natural foods, particularly lots of fresh fruit and vegetables.

In the third trimester
With a drop in your energy levels again due to the baby's increased growth, it's important to maintain a varied diet, eating smaller portions more often again.

After the birth
If breastfeeding, you'll need to increase your liquid intake and limit the amount of caffeine, alcohol and spicy food you consume (if any). Otherwise, simply maintain a healthy, diverse diet to support the body after birth.

Foods to enjoy:

Fruit: eat a maximum of three portions a day as fruit can be high in natural sugar; pineapple and papaya are great for digestion; apples, pears, apricots, nectarines, berries and avocado are easy to digest.

Vegetables: eat a wide range of vegetables to increase your vitamin and mineral intake; if suffering from digestive symptoms, limit vegetables such as cauliflower, cabbage, green peppers and tomatoes, which can be highly acidic.

Carbohydrates: rice (especially brown or red), sweet potatoes, pumpkin, oats, lentils and quinoa all release energy steadily and are easy to digest.

Protein: a moderate amount of thoroughly cooked (preferably organic) meat and poultry and/or eggs, beans, tofu and pulses will ensure you get enough protein to promote your baby's healthy growth.

Omega 3: eat a moderate amount of oily fish such as salmon and mackerel, which help with brain and nerve tissue development.

Dairy: eggs, milk, butter and hard cheeses can all be consumed in reasonable quantities to provide calcium for bone growth, but try to eat organic; dairy products can increase mucus in the body so limit your intake of this if experiencing colds or nasal swelling.

Foods to avoid:

Too much fruit: avoid excess fruit consumption and steer clear of bananas if constipated.

Wheat products: consume in moderation and eat only low processed varieties such as whole wheat bread or pasta.

Processed foods: limit or eliminate fizzy drinks, chocolates, biscuits, cakes and crisps, as they are low in nutrients and high in fat and salt, which can lead to excessive weight gain and water retention.

Preserved meats and smoked fish: consume in moderation as they are high in both salt and chemicals.

Certain fish: avoid tuna and swordfish as they can contain high levels of mercury; avoid raw shellfish.

Unpasteurised cheeses: avoid these as they can carry the bacteria Listeria.

Coffee or tea: drink in moderation or avoid completely as they affect the heart rate.

MOVING IN AND
OUT OF POSES

It is just as important to be aware of stability, balance, strength and flexibility as you move between yoga postures as it is to focus on these elements when holding any particular pose. Maintaining a stable base and moving slowly and evenly during every transition is particularly important when pregnant as you do not want to fall or jolt the baby in any way. Placing your attention on flowing between postures – rather than taking a stop-start approach – will help to keep your body safe and your mind focused.

From all fours to lying down

Start with your hands and feet apart in an all-fours (kneeling) position. Walk your right hand forwards and spread your fingers wide so that the hand can take more weight, and drop the elbow down.

Keeping your left hand closer to your body, turn to face the left side, walking your right knee towards the left and slowly lower your hips down, using your arm and hand strength until the one hip is secure on the floor.

Then move your right hand and arm towards your front and gently roll your right shoulder under and slowly roll onto your back.

From standing to all fours

Starting with your feet hip-width apart, place your hands on your knees, bend your knees deeply to allow your hips to sink down, and lean forwards.

Place one hand at a time on the floor, spreading your fingers and keeping your wrists under your shoulders.

Gently place one knee down at a time until you are secure on all fours.

Tip: It is particularly important that your pelvis remains stable if you suffer from symphysis pubis dysfunction (see p. 30) to prevent strain or pain. If you experience any pain in your hips during postures or moving from standing to sitting or kneeling positions, bring your knees and feet closer together to help to stabilise your pelvis.

THE IMPORTANCE OF GOOD BREATHING

By becoming aware of the breath within you – which flows, naturally and unrestricted, through your body – you'll learn how to be present in the moment and how to experience the universal life force (known in yogic terms as *prana*) that exists inside us all.

Enhancing breath control has a direct effect on calming the mind and creating a more positive outlook and, best of all, it will help to give your baby a rich blood supply to grow well.

There are many different yoga breathing techniques to encourage full use of the respiratory system, and these are particularly useful to practise during pregnancy as stress and strain on the body can affect posture and breathing ability.

Different breathing techniques have different benefits, whether calming or enhancing energy. As the ability to control your own breath increases, you will be more readily able to achieve your desired aims, and any accompanying visualisations will become more accessible and more potent.

As a beginner it can help to place your hands on the sides of your ribcage to bring awareness to how your body responds as you inhale and exhale. Imagine each time you inhale that the breath is making more space for your baby. Imagine each time you exhale that your baby feels more comfortable and secure in the womb.

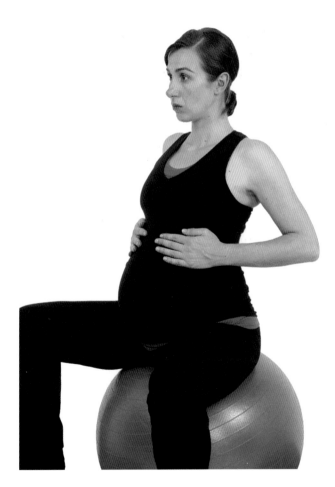

FULL YOGIC BREATHING

Taking a full yogic breath means using your lungs to their full capacity – inhaling maximum levels of oxygen and expelling maximum amounts of stale air. The full yogic breath accesses three areas of the lungs: the lower lungs near the abdomen, the thoracic area around the ribcage and the upper lungs near the chest. Practising full yogic breathing during pregnancy will help to create a feeling of freedom in the chest, which is especially important as the area gets more compressed in the later stages of pregnancy. Full breathing will also help to maintain high levels of oxygen – and therefore energy – in the body, which is important as you are now breathing for two.

1 Sit or lie in a comfortable position. Inhale and exhale naturally – in through the nose and out through the mouth – keeping your mind focused on the breathing action. This simple act is known as breath awareness. Let the breath flow in and out like a smooth, gentle wave, with no restrictions.

2 Take a slow, deep breath in, allowing the abdomen to gently expand and the diaphragm to press downwards. When the breath becomes fuller, let the ribcage expand until it feels like the spaces between the ribs are opening.

3 Once your lungs and chest feel fully expanded, take a slow, even breath out, allowing the abdomen to contract and the diaphragm to push upwards until the lungs are emptied.

This is one complete yogic breath. Practise this for a few minutes, or longer if it feels good.

Tip: Think of the lungs as big balloons that need to be blown up to their fullest before deflating back to their original size.

PELVIC BREATHING

Awareness of pelvic alignment is key to supporting your spine and abdomen as you go through the intense transformation that pregnancy brings about. The following 'pelvic breathing' exercises will create a stronger awareness of your pelvic base and its muscles, which will help to build confidence in being able to birth your baby with as much ease as possible. The exercises are best done after a sequence of other breathing techniques, or can be done after your posture practice when you are in a heightened state of awareness and ready to relax.

Tip: If you find sitting on the floor uncomfortable, sit on a pillow, lean against a wall, sit on a chair with your back supported or do the exercises standing, in Mountain pose.

1 Sit cross-legged on the floor or come into Butterfly (see p. 46).

2 As you inhale, lift your chest up, pull your shoulders blades down and in, gently tilt your pelvis back and feel your pelvic muscles slightly engage.

3 As you exhale, let your pelvis rock forwards, your chest and shoulders draw gently forwards and your pelvic muscles relax.

Repeat several times.

Variation: active pelvic breathing

1 Sit cross-legged or in Butterfly, place your hands on either side of your lower stomach.

2 As you exhale, gently push your hands into this area and feel the pressure change in your lower spine. At the end of your exhalation, aim to release all the tension from your lower back and relax your pelvic floor muscles.

3 Inhale, taking the pressure off your hands, then repeat the active exhalation again.

Repeat several times.

YOGA PROPS

Yoga is a relatively inexpensive exercise system to participate in as there is limited need for specialised equipment, other than a good quality yoga mat. However, a few simple extra props can give the body some much-needed extra help at times – especially during pregnancy.

Non-slip yoga mat
To stand, sit or lie on while you practise for comfort and grip. Mats come in different depths depending on how much cushion you want, but standard is usually 4–5mm (⅒–⅕ in) thick.

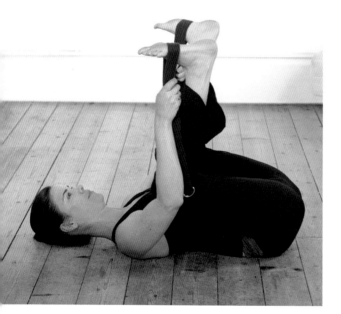

Strong wall
To lean against when full standing or sitting postures become too difficult.

Stable chair
To lean or sit on when full standing postures become too challenging (see p. 65 & p. 67 for examples of this in action).

Straps
To provide extra reach during stretching (see left and right), especially when your bump is getting in the way.

Blocks
To give support in certain postures, beneath your hands, hips or beneath your knees as in supported Butterfly (see far right), to support less flexible areas.

Cushions or pillows
To provide support where necessary for reclining and relaxation positions (see p. 82 & p. 128 for examples of this in action).

Bolsters

To offer support for relaxation, especially good under the knees when lying down (see p. 128).

Exercise ball

To sit on towards the later stages of pregnancy when it can be uncomfortable to do seated postures on a more rigid surface (see p. 73 & p. 91 for examples of this in action). Also useful when performing Hip Rolls (see p. 48) or Wide-leg Seated Stretches (see pp. 94–97), due to its curves.

Blankets

To support your neck and hips when folded beneath them, and to keep you warm during final relaxation.

Eye mask

To encourage sense withdrawal and therefore maximum relaxation.

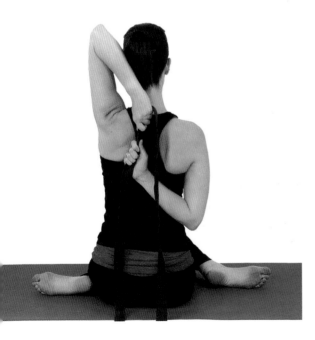

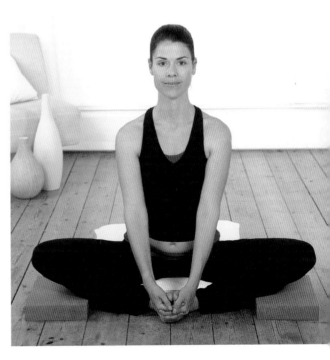

MODIFICATIONS

During pregnancy, women can experience strong physical symptoms that create discomfort in the body and can make physical activities more difficult. With a few special modifications, you can often continue with your yoga practice and, in many cases, the modified exercises may even help to alleviate your symptoms. It's always best, however, to check with a medical expert first.

Symphysis Pubis Dysfunction (SPD)

A condition that causes excess movement in the pelvis. The main symptom is usually pain or discomfort in the pelvic area.

When you practise yoga with SPD, heightened focus should be placed on creating stability in the pelvis. Strive for slow, purposeful movements that encourage bone and joint stacking through proper alignment. Avoid deep squats, wide leg stretches, strong twisting movements and deep lunges.

Carpal Tunnel Syndrome

This occurs when the median nerve, which runs from the forearm into the palm, becomes squeezed at the wrist. The result may be pain, weakness or numbness in the hand and wrist, radiating up the arm.

When doing any postures that require pressure on the palms, try to either cup the palms or make fists and place the top of the fists on the floor. Work on strengthening your grip by regularly squeezing a tennis ball.

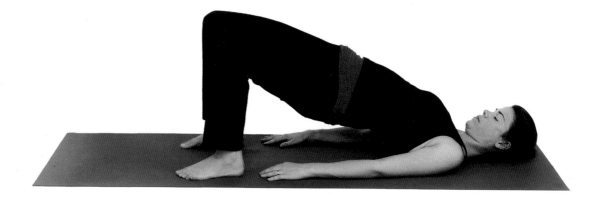

Sciatica

This condition is caused by pressure on the sciatic nerve, which comes from your lower back, travels down the back of your legs and branches out to your feet. The pressure is usually a result of a compressed lumbar disc in the area of the nerve. Symptoms can be pins and needles, or acute pain.

Try to limit any postures where the leg is lifted up in front of you. When bending forwards, keep your knees bent and the spine straight. Avoid sitting for long periods of time. And do postures such as Cowface (see p. 54) and Bridge (see p. 56) that help to stabilise the pelvic floor and tone the lower back and stomach muscles.

Restless Leg Syndrome (RLS)

This nervous system disorder creates a need to move the legs to stop unpleasant sensations. The symptoms are often felt most acutely at night, which means RLS is also considered a sleep disorder.

Exercises such as Cat (see p. 52) with calf stretches and bicycle legs in Downward Dog position (see p. 36) will help to maintain healthy circulation in the legs, while those such as Legs Up the Wall (see right) and Shoulderstand (see p. 58) can help to relax the legs. Breathing practices and relaxation techniques will help to counteract the lack of good sleep.

Low-lying Placenta

This condition occurs when the placenta is in a low-lying position covering the cervix, rather than the normal higher position, on the inside wall of the uterus. Symptoms can include vaginal bleeding, especially later in the pregnancy, and labour-type pains.

Avoid deep squats, wide leg stretches and deep lunges. Always practise gently and be sure to modify postures using chairs and other supports where necessary.

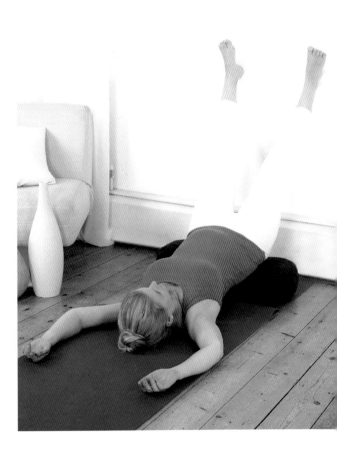

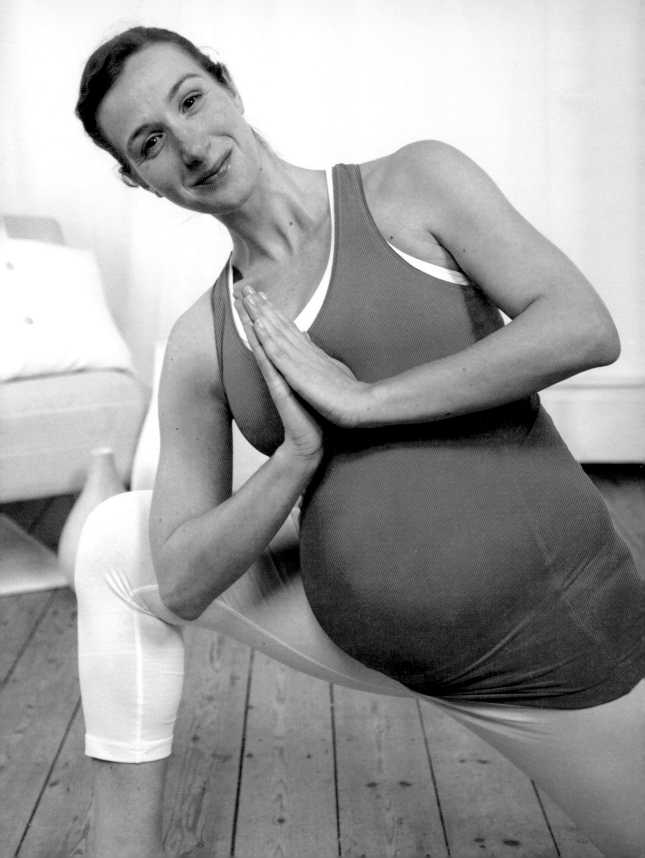

WARM-UP

The nurturing Sun Salutation sequence on the pages that follow has been specially adapted for pregnancy. You can do several rounds of it at the start of a yoga practice to warm you up or as a full session in its own right.

For a slower, meditative practice, hold each posture for several breaths before moving on to the next one. This is ideal if you are new to yoga, feel a little lacking in energy or simply feel like your body needs to take its time.

Alternatively, for a more dynamic practice, try moving between postures with the flow of your breath. This will enhance energy, build strength and flexibility, as well as deepening the mind-body connection.

Whichever approach you take, be sure to remain aware of natural, changing energy levels and always take things down a notch when needed. Begin your practice slowly with a couple of rounds of the sequence. Then, as you gain experience and familiarity, work up to six rounds, assuming Child's pose (see p. 122) if you need to rest between, or during, rounds. If you want to challenge yourself a little more with an extended sequence, the additional postures on pages 40–43 can be inserted into the basic sequence.

BASIC SUN SALUTATION SEQUENCE

The Sun Salutation sequence is a great way to warm up your body – stretching, toning and invigorating you all over. It is important to maintain a steady rhythm throughout, regardless of whether that is fast or slow. Remember that at any point you can rest in Child's pose (see p. 122). This is especially important in the first and third trimester when your body can be easily fatigued and is more vulnerable.

Mountain pose

1 Stand with your feet hip-width apart and parallel, your heels directly behind your toes.

2 Distribute your weight equally over both feet and bend your knees slightly.

✳ **Tip:** Mountain pose is the foundation for all other postures so it's important to practise it with proper alignment, extension and awareness. It is a great tool at any time for checking correct alignment in the whole body, which is particularly important to do as your posture shifts during pregnancy.

3 Lengthen your spine upwards through the crown of your head, and open the front side of your body, expanding your chest and lifting your diaphragm as you pull your shoulders back and down.

4 Drop your chin down slightly to lengthen and open the back of your neck.

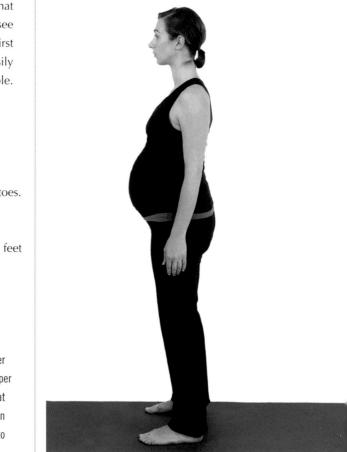

5 Allow your arms to hang free, with thumbs turned out slightly to bring the inner crease of your elbows to face forwards. Palms should face into your thighs.

6 Gently tuck your tailbone under and contract your buttocks. This will help to engage the pelvic floor and create more lift through the torso.

7 Relax your face and jaw, become still and steady, and breathe naturally.

Mountain pose with raised arms

8 Standing in Mountain pose, exhale to centre yourself, inhale and slowly raise your arms over your head, keeping your shoulders gently pulled down and your hands shoulder-width apart. Stretch up through your fingers and down through your heels. Your arms should feel like an extension of your spine.

9 Exhale, bend your knees to squat deeply and bring your arms down by your sides, fingertips reaching to the floor. Walk your hands forwards on the floor.

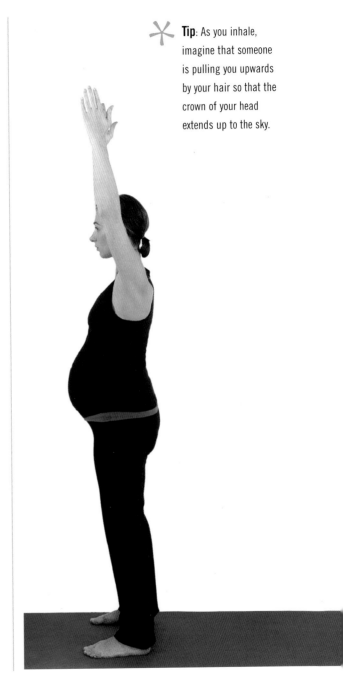

Tip: As you inhale, imagine that someone is pulling you upwards by your hair so that the crown of your head extends up to the sky.

Downward dog

10 Gently come into a kneeling tabletop position. Place your hands under your shoulders with your fingers spread wide, knees under your hips and toes tucked under so that feet are flexed.

11 Pull your shoulders back to make space in your chest and upper back, and breathe naturally.

12 If feeling strong, exhale and press firmly with your palms into the floor, straightening your legs and lifting your sitting bones up as high as possible. Aim to eventually straighten your legs fully and press your heels down into the floor.

Tip: If your neck and shoulders are stiff, turn your palms and fingers slightly outwards. If the above posture feels too strong, try the kneeling variation described in step 10.

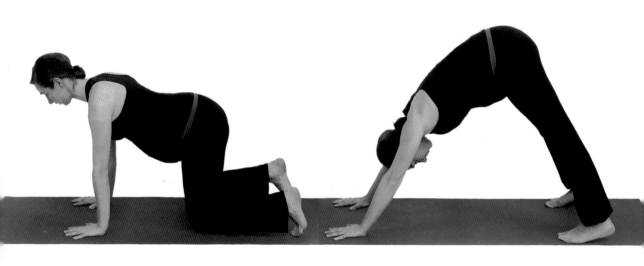

Gentle plank

13   Gently come into a kneeling tabletop position. Walk your hands forwards about 15cm (6in). Point your toes backwards, so the top of your feet are flat on the floor.

14   Inhale and gently engage your stomach muscles, then shift your body forwards so that your shoulders are directly over your hands and your back is almost horizontal. Pull your shoulders back and down to maintain space in your chest and upper back.

15   Only hold this position briefly, breathing comfortably, before coming back to tabletop position, on all fours.

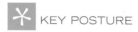
Child's pose

16 From a kneeling tabletop position, turn your knees outwards and bring your big toes together.

17 Exhale and shift your hips backwards until they rest on your heels. Your baby bump should rest nicely between your legs. Relax your neck and let your forehead rest gently on the floor.

18 Inhale and feel your chest and lungs expand. Exhale and walk your fingers forwards until you feel a long, deep opening down the front of your body.

Tip: Child's pose is one of the best relaxation postures and can be practised at any point if you need to rest. By resting your head below the level of your heart, your breath and heart rate slow down, allowing muscles, joints and major stress points to relax. It is a great posture to practise before bed, especially if your mind is racing with thoughts, as it will help to calm you down. To adapt the posture as you progress through your pregnancy, widen your knees and use pillows under your head and chest for support to accommodate your growing baby. You should always feel relaxed in this posture.

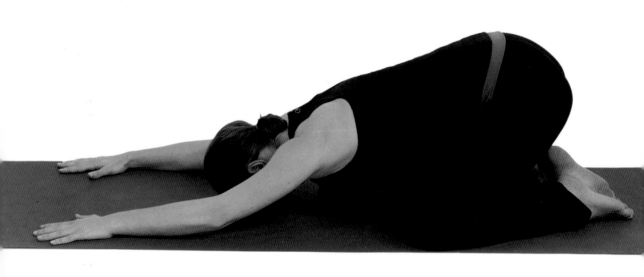

Downward dog

19 Inhale and bring your body into tabletop position, on all fours. Hands in line with shoulders and knees directly under the hips, with feet extended backwards.

20 If feeling strong, exhale, tuck your toes under, press your palms firmly into the floor and aim to straighten your legs. Try to create maximum space through your spine as you lift your sitting bones upwards. Hold for several breaths.

Mountain pose with hands in prayer

21 From Downward Dog, gently bend your knees and walk your feet forwards.

22 Keeping your knees and feet wide and feet firmly planted, inhale and slowly stand upright, placing your hands on your thighs for support if necessary. As you become more upright, raise your arms out and up until your palms meet overhead – in *anjali mudra*, or Prayer position. Then exhale and bring your hands, still in prayer, down to your chest.

23 Breathe and enjoy feeling centred – calm but energised.

EXTENDED SEQUENCE

After getting used to the basic Sun Salutation sequence and being able to comfortably practise several rounds, you may wish to start adding in extra postures for more of a stronger practice. Each of the four postures that follow can be slotted in individually to follow Child's pose (see p. 38) and then practised sequentially as a flowing sequence when you are more familiar with the postures and the order.

Tip: If this feels too strong, practise this leg extension from a tabletop position. Do not practise if you have SPD (see p. 30).

Downward dog with leg extension

1 From Child's pose, inhale and come forward onto all fours, tuck your toes under, inhale and lift into Downward Dog (see p. 36).

2 Press your hands and feet firmly down to create stability, inhale and lift your right leg straight back and up. Keep your foot flexed and stretch back into your heel. Hold for several comfortable breaths.

3 Exhale and bring your leg down, or gracefully move straight into Gentle Lunge at step 2. Repeat on the other side. Note that as your bump gets bigger, the hip of the raised leg can lift higher to create more space, but always try to keep the shoulders square.

Gentle lunge

1 From Child's pose, gently come into a kneeling tabletop position.

2 Inhale and bring your right foot forward so that it is on the outside of your right hand.

3 Exhale and gently push your right hip down to open the lower back and hip areas. Hold for several breaths. Reverse slowly back to tabletop position and repeat on the other side.

4 If feeling strong while in each lunge, walk your front foot in a little towards the centre, press your foot firmly down, inhale and lift your body upright, placing your hands on your front thigh to stabilise yourself. If comfortable here, raise one or both of your arms overhead. Hold for several comfortable breaths.

5 Exhale and slowly reverse out.

Tip: If you're struggling with balance, try doing this posture with a chair beside you, placing one hand on it for stability.

Gentle prayer twist

1 From Gentle Lunge (see p. 41), on your right leg, bring your hands together into Prayer position in front of your chest, keeping your shoulders down and elbows tucked into your body.

2 Inhale and open your chest. Exhale and twist to your left side, placing your right elbow to the inside of your right knee. Hold for several comfortable breaths.

3 Inhale and slowly untwist to the front, release your hands to your right thigh, then slowly place your hands on the floor to the inside of your leg.

4 Release to all fours, Child's pose or Downward Dog. Repeat on the other side, with your left leg forward in the lunge.

✳ **Tip**: Only perform this posture if you're feeling strong and stable.

Gentle side plank

1 Gently come into a kneeling tabletop position.

2 Inhale, turn your right foot and lower leg sideways to keep your body stable in the posture. Extend your left leg straight back and try to press the outside of your left foot into the floor with the foot in a flexed angle. At the same time, gently push both hips forwards.

3 Use your right hand, right knee and left foot for support as you inhale and stretch your left arm directly upwards trying to create space in the chest and between the shoulders.

4 Turn the palm to face forward, inhale and stretch the arm over your left ear. Hold for several comfortable breaths.

5 Exhale and bring your left hand to the floor and return to kneeling tabletop position.

Repeat on the other side.

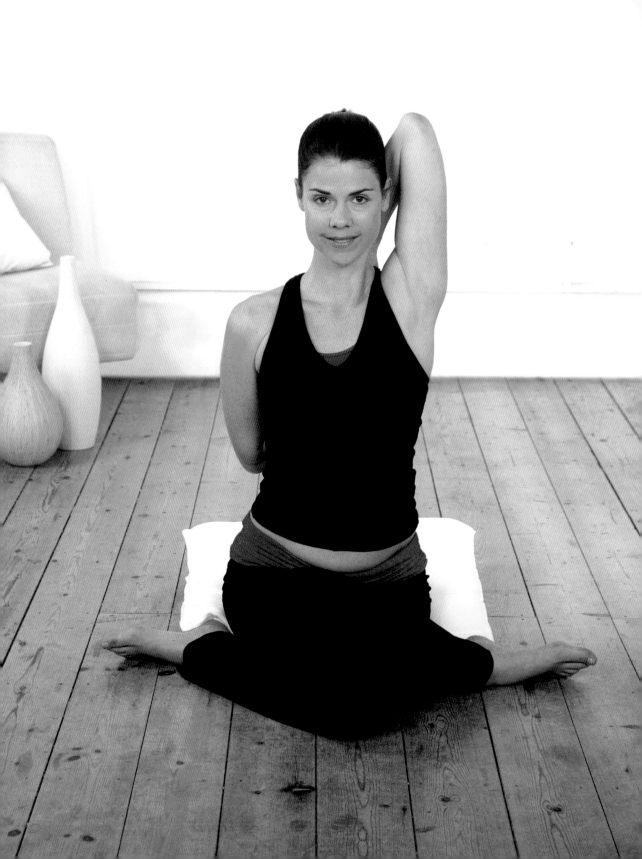

FIRST TRIMESTER POSTURES

The first trimester of your pregnancy is a time to focus on accepting change, nurturing yourself and building strength to support your unborn child. As hormones are strong, your emotions and energy levels are probably shifting dramatically, so go slow, breathe deeply and aim to set strong foundations for a yoga practice that will carry you through the rest of your pregnancy.

You can practise the postures in the following pages at any time during your first trimester, choosing the most appropriate variation of each one to suit your ever-changing needs.

Just be sure to do a few rounds of Sun Salutation (see pp. 34–39) first to get your body warmed up beforehand. And remember to practise relaxation poses (see pp. 120–129) at any time you feel the need and especially afterwards to unwind and really reap the benefits from the physical work that you have done.

BUTTERFLY

Many people are surprised how tight their hips feel when they try this pose for the first time. Spending a lot of time sitting in a chair tightens the ligaments and muscles around your hips, as well as making your knees stiff. Practising Butterfly from this early stage of pregnancy will bring increased flexibility to these areas, which will be a great advantage during the birth of your baby.

1   Sit in an upright position on the floor. Place your hands behind you for support, bend your knees, bring the soles of your feet together and let your knees open outwards, so your legs are in a diamond shape.

2   Press into your palms and soles of the feet, inhale and gently lift your hips forward towards your heels until you feel a stretch, but never overstrain! Walk your hands forwards and sit up. Lean forwards, interlace your fingers under both feet, pressing your soles together.

3   Inhale, stretch your spine upwards and let your knees gently press downwards. Relax and gently flap your knees several times like a butterfly's wings.

4   To deepen the stretch, exhale and lean gently forwards, pressing your knees down and outwards. Hold for several comfortable breaths at your deepest stretch, then release as you inhale. Repeat again.

5   To soften your hips and pelvis, maintain the Butterfly position and gently rock from side to side for about 20 seconds.

Tip: If your knees are extremely stiff, place pillows, cushions or blocks under them so that you don't strain the ligaments of your groin. Remember, never overstretch!

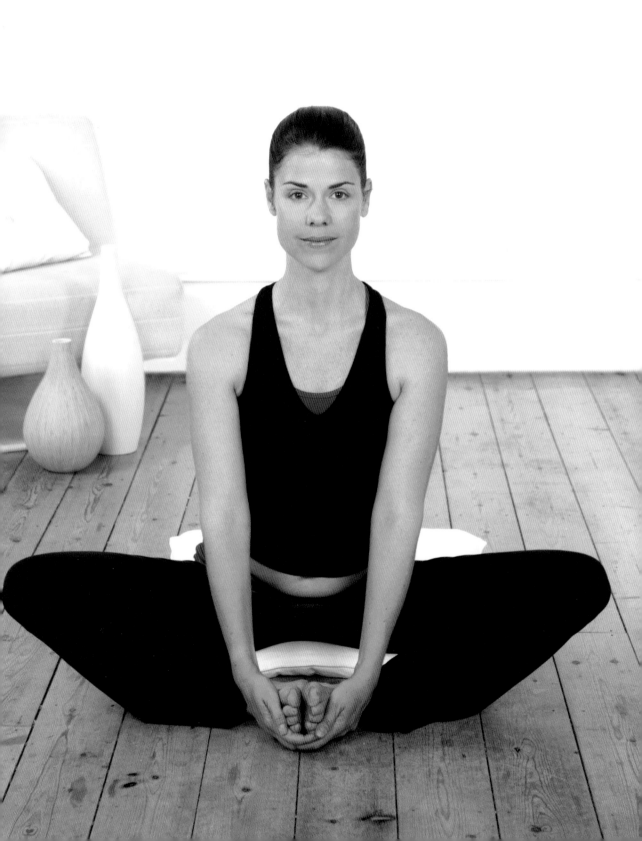

HIP ROLLS I

This forward-backward hip motion will help to release tension from your hips and lower back, as well as bringing heightened awareness to your pelvic muscles. It is therefore great to do throughout your pregnancy in preparation for labour.

1 Sit upright in Butterfly (see p. 46), resting on the edge of a cushion or folded blanket for comfort if desired. Place your hands about 25cm (10in) behind you on the floor, with your fingers turned outwards.

2 Inhale and lift your chest up, pull your shoulders back and down, let your pelvis tilt back so you feel the sitting bones press back and down, and gently engage your stomach and pelvic muscles.

3 Exhale and let your pelvis rock forwards, gently draw your chest and shoulders forwards and relax your pelvic muscles. Repeat several times.

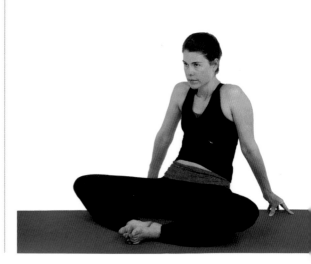

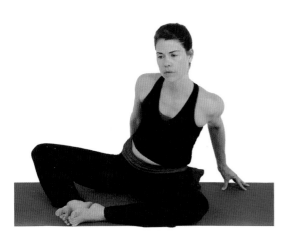

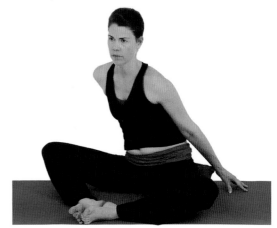

HIP ROLLS II

The circular hip motion involved in this posture
really opens your hips and pelvic area, helping
you to work through any areas of tightness and
increase overall flexibility. Be sure to
breathe deeply as you move through the
hip rolls to support the movement.

1 Sit upright in Butterfly (see p. 46), resting
on the edge of a cushion or folded blanket
for comfort if desired. Place your hands
12–15cm (5–6in) behind you on the floor,
with your fingers turned outwards.

✳ **Tip**: If sitting on a rigid surface becomes
uncomfortable, you could try these postures
on an exercise ball, kneeling or standing
with your hands against a wall.

2 Relax your hips so your pelvis is tilted under.
Your shoulders will be slightly lifted upwards
to begin with.

3 Inhale and move your upper body to the left
as your hips rock to the right. Then move
slowly in a clockwise direction so that, at
the height of your inhalation, your chest is
forwards and your pelvis tilting backwards,
keeping your shoulders down.

4 Exhale and move your upper body to the
right, as your hips rock to the left. Continue
to move in a clockwise direction so that, at
the height of your exhalation, you are back
at the point where you began.

Repeat three times in total. Then repeat three
times in the opposite direction.

EAGLE ARMS

The shoulders and neck are often areas that hold a lot stress. This strong shoulder-opening posture will help you to release this stress and therefore feel more in control as you undergo the changes that pregnancy brings. It can be done at any time – either standing, kneeling, leaning against a wall or sitting.

1 Sit upright in a cross-legged position, lift your arms straight out in front of you and bring your left arm underneath your right arm, crossing at the elbows.

2 Bend your arms so that your fingers point upwards, cross your arms again at the wrists and aim to press your palms together, so that your thumbs are closest to your body and little fingers furthest away. You can try to make your wrists straighter by interlacing your fingers and then opening the fingers out and pressing the palms together.

3 As you gently breathe in and out, pull your elbows down, then stretch them upwards, feeling the different effect on the shoulders. Repeat for several breaths and release.

Repeat on the other side.

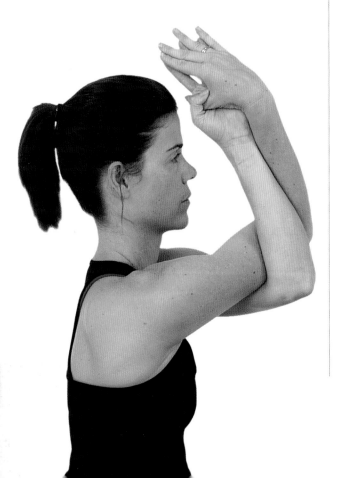

FINGERS INTERLACED

Stretching your hands above your head in this posture helps to release any tension in your shoulders and neck. Stretching to the side then provides a welcome sense of opening down each side of your body, promoting an increased sense of lightness.

1 Sit in a cross-legged position and place your hands in your lap, fingers interlaced. Inhale and raise your arms upwards, knuckles up, stretching up through your spine, arms, neck and the backs of your hands, and keeping your shoulders down. Exhale and slowly lower your arms. Repeat several times.

2 Bring your hands to Prayer position (*anjali mudra*, see p. 39) in front of your chest and interlace your fingers (and thumbs) but release your index fingers so that they press against each other. Keeping your hands in this position, inhale and stretch your arms overhead, elbows close to your ears.

3 Exhale and slowly stretch your arms to the left, holding for several comfortable breaths. Repeat to the right, then exhale and lower arms down through the centre.

Repeat steps 3–5 several times.

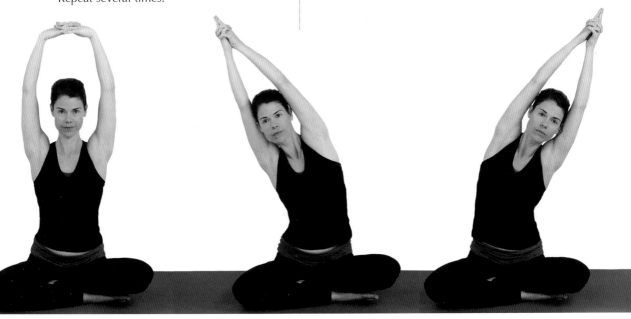

CAT

The Cat pose is fantastic for alleviating tension in the back, neck and shoulders, and for helping to keep pelvic muscles toned, supple and stable. As well as being a valuable posture in its own right, the neutral starting position of Cat pose can be used as a stable transition pose or when stronger standing postures are too difficult.

1 Kneel on all fours in a tabletop position, with your knees directly under your hips and your wrists under shoulders. Palms should be flat on the floor and fingers spread out, with index fingers pointing forwards. Your spine should feel long.

2 Inhale and ensure your shoulders are down (not hunched). Exhale and tilt your pelvis inwards and under, engaging your pelvic muscles while tucking your chin in. This should create a curve (opening) on your back. For an increased stretch, raise yourself up on your fingertips.

3 Inhale and gently tilt your pelvis back, lift your head up and return your spine to a neutral position.

Repeat several times.

Cat variations

The following variations from Cat pose are fun, safe and provide added benefits:

Calf stretch: From tabletop position on all fours, straighten your right leg behind you, tuck the toes under so the foot is flexed with toes resting on the floor. Inhale, gently stretch your heel away from you. Hold for several comfortable breaths. Repeat on the left leg.

Raised-leg push-up: From a tabletop position on all fours, exhale and extend your right leg behind you. Inhale, then as you exhale, bend your elbows to bring your chest to elbow-height, raising your leg up so that your spine and leg are in a straight line. Inhale, push your upper body upwards and gently lower your leg back to kneeling. Repeat several times on each side, building up repetitions as you get stronger.

Upper back twist (see below): From tabletop position on all fours, lower yourself gently onto your elbows, inhale and raise your right arm directly upwards, turning your upper body to the right so that both shoulders come into one line. Extend as far as you can and hold for several comfortable breaths. Then exhale and release your arm down. Repeat on the other side.

COWFACE

This pose helps to stretch your hamstrings and the outside of your hips and buttocks, as well as relieving pressure around your back and opening your chest, shoulders and arms. It is therefore good to practise in the first trimester when your bust and bump are smaller – and throughout the rest of your pregnancy if you enjoy the benefits.

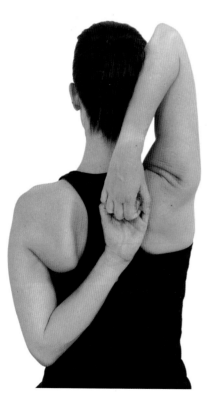

1 Sit in a cross-legged, upright position, place your hands about 20cm (8in) behind you and lean backwards.

2 Lift your right leg and place your foot flat on the floor in front of you so that your knee points upwards. Gently move your left knee and heel to the right, so that your left knee, still on the floor, is pointing directly forwards, in line with your groin, and your left heel is on the outside of your right hip.

3 Lean forwards and use your left hand to gently move your right foot and leg towards the outside of your left knee, allowing your right knee to lower on top of your left one so that they become stacked in the centre. Your right ankle should rest on the floor, close to your left hip.

4 With stable hips, sit upright, inhale and raise your left arm up above your head. Bend your elbow so that it points towards the ceiling while your left hand rests on your back, palm inwards.

5 Inhale, bring your right arm behind your lower back and bend the elbow so it points downwards, fingers pointing upwards, palm facing out. Exhale and gently walk your

hands together until they meet; if they meet, clasp your fingers.

6 Inhale, open your chest and bring your top elbow further back so that it sits behind your head. Hold for several breaths, then release.

Repeat on the other side.

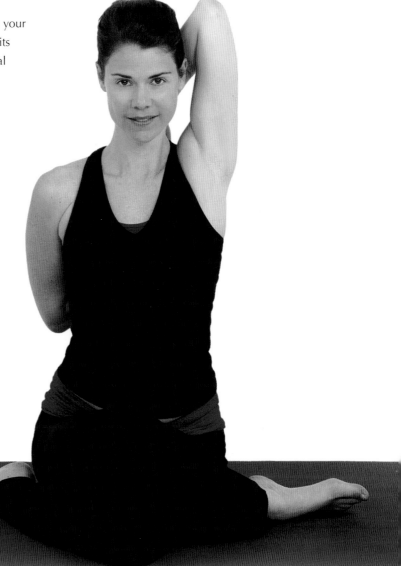

Tip: If your hands don't meet behind your back, try using a yoga strap (see pp. 28–29) between them until you become more flexible.

BRIDGE

This is a gentle back bend that helps to strengthen and stretch your back and abdominal muscles. It is also good for stimulating the thyroid gland, which can become unbalanced in pregnancy. Practising this pose will therefore help to regulate your metabolism.

1 Lie on your back, with your arms close to your body, palms facing downwards. Bend your legs so that your feet are planted flat on the floor, hip-width apart, and your knees are directly above your heels, toes pointing forwards.

2 Inhale, then exhale and slowly raise your hips and upper back towards the ceiling. Exhale and interlace your fingers, keeping your arms on the floor.

Tip: As you press your chin into your throat, think about making a double chin. This chin lock is what helps to stimulate and regulate the thyroid gland.

3 Inhale, raise your chest and pull your shoulders down. Gently press your chin down to lengthen your neck and form a slight chin lock. Hold for several breaths, focusing on the opening of your front and your pelvic floor, before you exhale and release.

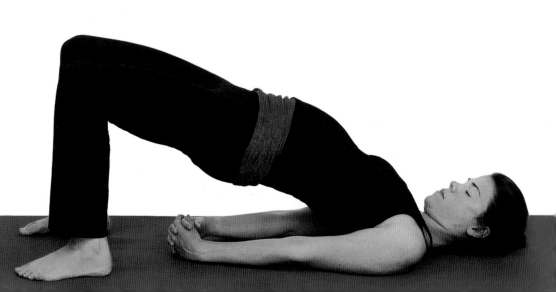

BRIDGE WITH HIP MOVEMENTS

This gentle series of Bridge movements will help to build pelvic awareness and strength in preparation for your baby's development, which is particularly important in the first trimester when the pelvis is still relatively stable.

1 Lie on your back, with your knees bent, your feet flat on the floor directly under your knees and your arms relaxed by your sides.

2 As you exhale, press your middle back down into the floor so that your pelvis tilts slightly, inhale and relax. Repeat several times.

3 Gently lift your hips off the floor and rock them side-to-side.

4 Keeping your hips in the air, make first several clockwise circles with your hips, then several counterclockwise ones, while breathing comfortably.

5 If you are feeling strong, inhale and lift your hips higher, exhale and drop your left hip down, as you raise the right hip up. Remember to keep both shoulders stable, pressing into the floor. Hold for several breaths, then repeat on the opposite side.

6 Exhale, relax your hips down and release your legs to Butterfly (see p. 46), or fully extend them to Corpse pose (see p. 128).

Tip: Be aware of whether one hip feels tighter than the other and see if this imbalance changes over time.

SHOULDERSTAND

Less intense than the regular, fully inverted Shoulderstand, this specially adapted variation is ideal for pregnancy. You will still get all the same benefits of releasing pressure on your legs, back and hips, improving circulation to your legs and pelvis, and relaxing both your body and your mind.

1 Gently lie on your back, close to a stable wall and lift your legs up onto the wall. Press your feet into the wall, lift your hips a little and position a large cushion or bolster under your hips in a comfortable spot.

2 Fully relax your head, neck and shoulders into the floor with palms facing downwards. Breathe deeply and relax.

3 Exhale, press your back into the support, raise your hips and straighten your legs and stretch through to your heels.

4 Inhale and stretch your arms above your head on the floor. As you breathe, keep extending the stretch. Release your arms to their original position, by the body, after several breaths.

5 If you are comfortable with this and feeling strong, inhale, push your feet firmly into the wall and, keeping your knees bent, press your hips forwards, so you have a slight chin lock and your back is relatively straight. Hold for several comfortable breaths, then release.

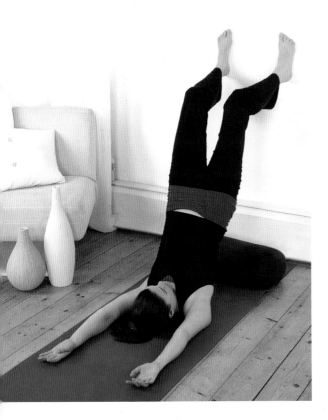

 Tip: Make sure that you have a bolster or large cushion available for this posture.

FISH POSE

Due to the chin lock and compression experienced in Bridge (see p. 56) and Shoulderstand (opposite) it is important to counteract them with an extension posture like Fish pose. This stretches the throat and chest passages, which helps to promote easier breathing. It also helps to stimulate the thyroid gland, which is good for regulating metabolism and energy levels. Plus it is a great restorative pose at any time to counteract negative emotions.

Tip: Avoid this pose if you have heart problems or any serious back conditions.

1 Lie on your back, with your arms close to your body, palms downwards, feet planted flat, hip-width apart, and knees directly above your heels, toes pointing forwards.

2 Place a rolled towel, blanket or bolster lengthways under your middle back.

3 Exhale, then inhale and arch your back aiming to gently rest the crown of your head on the floor, using your back muscles and elbows to support the arch and lift of your spine.

4 If comfortable here, let your knees gently open to the sides in Butterfly (see p. 46). Blocks or supports can be placed under your knees for comfort if needed. Inhale and expand your chest fully and let the throat open. Exhale and relax your hips, pelvis and lower back. Hold for several breaths.

5 Gently raise your knees back up, with weight on your elbows, and slowly release your head. Remove the back support, extend your legs, lie flat and relax deeply.

HAPPY BABY

This posture is so-called as your baby will naturally start doing it at around four or five months old. Practising the pose yourself will create a sense of opening in your hip and pelvic area as well as helping to release pressure from your lower back and opening your chest.

1 Lie on your back, gently bend your knees and lift them to either side of your torso.

2 Inhale and grip the outsides of your feet with your hands, five fingers together.

3 Exhale and gently pull on your feet to bring your knees downwards, shins directly over your knees. Gently flexing your feet and pushing them upwards, as if you are standing on the ceiling, will help to create some resistance.

4 As you breathe in this position, let your tailbone extend, your shoulders drop down into the floor and your neck lengthen. Hold for several comfortable breaths, then release.

Tip: If it is difficult to reach the outside of your feet, place a yoga strap or towel around each foot and hold the ends with each hand.

HAPPY BABY
ON SIDE

Happy Baby on your side can be practised as a gentle rolling extension of the main pose at this early stage of pregnancy or individually in the later stages, when it is difficult to lie on your back. When done as a gentle flow from Happy Baby, remember to transition slowly, using your breath as a guide. This will allow for greater safety, hip-opening and lower back loosening.

1   Lie down on your left side. Extend your left arm and rest your head on it. Keep your left knee slightly bent and the fingers of your right hand on the floor in front so you feel comfortable and stable.

2   Inhale, take hold of your right leg just below the knee with your right hand and raise your right knee upwards, towards your body.

3   Exhale and pull your knee gently towards your right armpit and hold for a few seconds. Ensure your shoulder is pulled down and your elbow is tucked in.

4   Exhale and release before gently rolling onto your back and onto the other side to repeat.

Do the sequence twice in total.

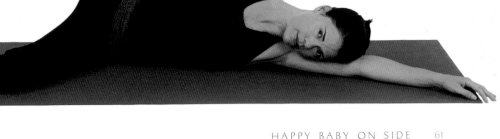

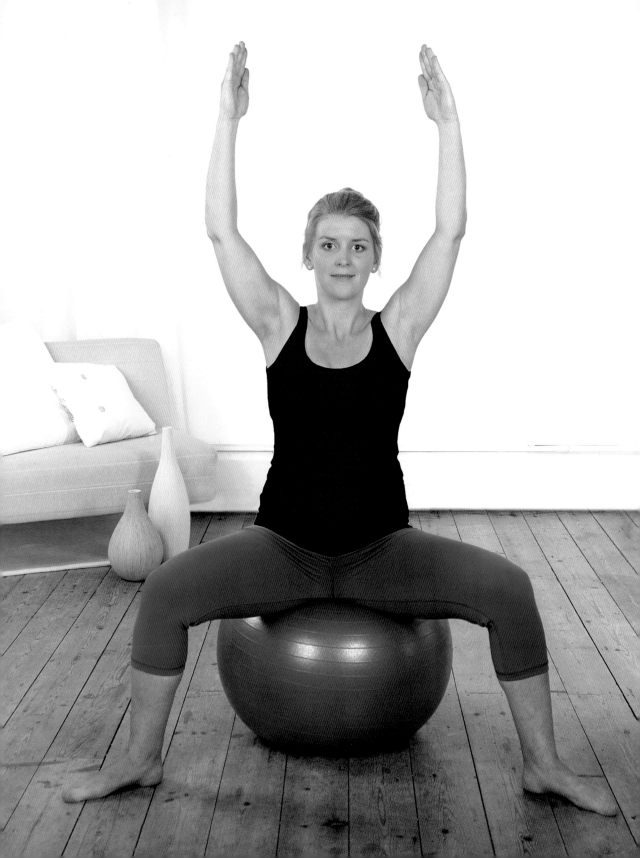

SECOND TRIMESTER POSTURES

The second trimester of your pregnancy is when the strong hormone shifts start to alleviate and you start to feel more balanced. As a result, you are likely to experience a surge in energy and positivity. Finally, you can start to really enjoy your pregnancy! As your body and mind feel more stable, this is a great time to build strength and stamina in your yoga practice.

You can practise the postures in the following pages at any time during your second trimester, choosing the most appropriate variation of each one to suit your ever-changing needs. Just be sure to do a few rounds of Sun Salutation (see pp. 34–39) to get the body well warmed up beforehand, and take time to practise relaxation poses afterwards to unwind.

Also remember that although the second trimester is generally a time of increased energy, it is still important to rest any time you feel tired.

WARRIOR II

The Warrior postures help to build strength, confidence and stamina. They can be quite powerful if you are new to yoga, so begin by trying the supported versions, where you can focus on proper alignment. Then, once you feel stronger, you can try them unsupported. Warrior II, which is particularly useful for external hip-opening, is presented before Warrior I in the following sequence as many people find the hip position easier to attain than the internal hip rotation of Warrior I.

1 Start in a strong, wide-legged stance, feet parallel. Place your hands on your hips, inhale and stretch your spine upwards.

2 Turn your left foot out to the side and move your right foot out a little to widen the stance further, positioning it to face forwards, at a 90-degree angle to your left foot. Keep your hips facing forwards and your shoulders down.

3 Exhale and bend your left knee, keeping it directly over your ankle as you lower your hips.

4 Inhale and raise both arms out to shoulder-height, with fingers extended, and look straight ahead or towards your left arm if your neck feels comfortable. Hold for three breaths, then release.

Repeat on the other side.

Variation: supported

1 Sit comfortably, facing forwards, on the edge of a sturdy chair with your legs wide open and feet flat on the floor, angled outwards for stability. Rest your hands on your hips, inhale and lengthen your spine upwards with your shoulders down.

2 Exhale, turn your left foot out to the side and straighten your right leg, positioning your right foot to face forwards, at a 90-degree angle to your left foot. Keep both hips pointing forwards and the spine straight.

3 Inhale and raise both arms out to shoulder-height, with fingers extended, and look straight ahead or towards your left arm if your neck feels comfortable. Hold for three breaths, then release.

Repeat on the other side to complete one cycle Build up to two or three cycles to build strength and stamina.

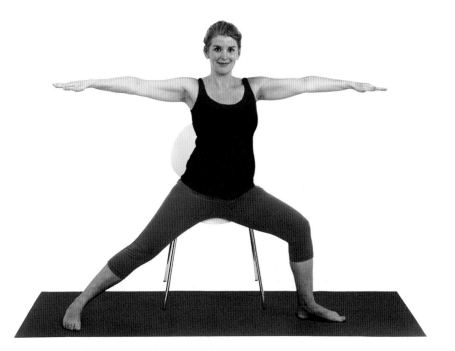

WARRIOR I

Warrior I differs from Warrior II in that the hips are rotated in the direction of the front foot, which creates a greater sense of opening for the hip flexors, calves, ankles, chest and sides. The pose will also strengthen your thighs, creating a stable lower body foundation to support the increased weight of the baby.

1 Start in a strong, wide-legged stance, feet parallel. Place your hands on your hips, inhale and stretch your spine upwards.

2 Turn your left foot out to the side, move your right foot out a little to widen the stance further, and position your right foot at a 60-degree angle to your left one. Turn your hips and chest to face the the same direction as your left foot.

3 Exhale and bend your left knee, keeping your knee directly over your ankle as you lower your hips.

4 Inhale and raise both arms upwards, keeping hands shoulder-width apart, and hold for three breaths.

5 Exhale and bring your arms down, placing your hands on your hips, and release.

Repeat on the opposite side to complete one cycle. Build up to two or three cycles to build strength and stamina.

Variation: supported

1 Sit comfortably on the edge of a sturdy chair with your legs wide open and feet angled outwards for stability. Place your hands on your hips, inhale and lengthen your spine upwards, keeping your shoulders down.

2 Exhale, turn your left foot out to the side and straighten your right leg out to the side, positioning your right foot at a 60-degree angle to your left one. Turn your hips and chest in the same direction as your left foot, placing your hands on your hips.

3 Inhale and lift both arms upwards, keeping hands shoulder-width apart. Exhale and press the outside of your right foot into the floor. Hold for three breaths.

4 Exhale and bring your arms down, placing your hands on your hips, and release.

Repeat on the opposite side to complete one cycle. Build up to two or three cycles when feeling strong.

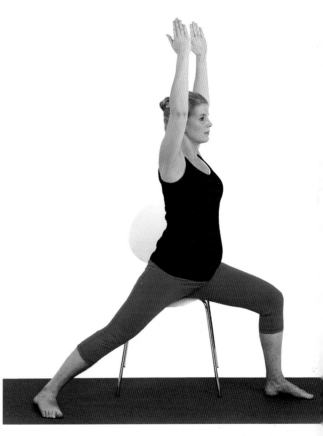

TRIANGLE

The Triangle posture is a classic yoga position that stretches your spine, inner thigh, abdominal and side muscles. It also helps to open the pelvis by stretching the pelvic ligaments but be careful to practise slowly and with awareness. As the baby bump gets bigger this is a great posture to help create space and openness in the body.

1 Stand with your legs over a metre (3 feet) apart, with your feet pointed forwards and your hands on your hips. Then turn your left foot out to point to the side and push your hips gently forwards, keeping your spine straight.

2 Inhale and lift both arms out to shoulder-height. Exhale and bend your body to the

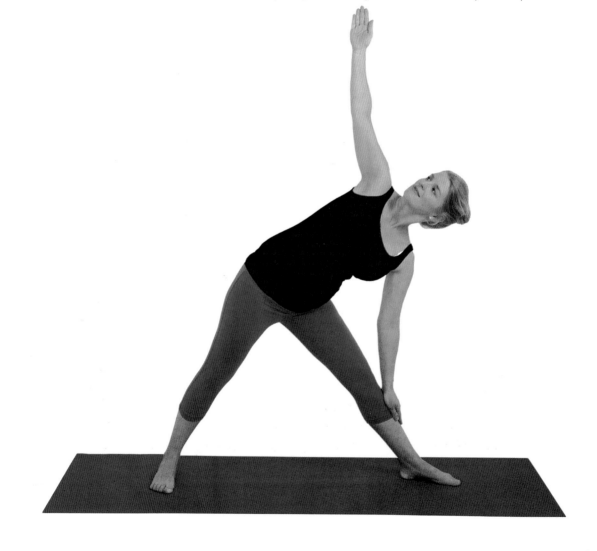

left, placing your left hand on your left shin, or higher if needed. Inhale and bring your right hand to rest on your lower back, pulling your shoulder backwards to open and rotate your chest.

3 If both shoulders are in line and you feel stable, inhale and raise your right arm upwards. Hold for several comfortable breaths, then reverse out of the pose.

Repeat on the other side.

Variation: supported

1 Stand with a sturdy chair on your left, about a metre (3 feet) away. Place your hands on your hips, lift your left leg up and place your foot, turned 90-degree outwards, on the seat of the chair. Both legs should be straight.

2 Gently push both hips forwards, keeping your shoulders directly over your hips. Inhale, then exhale and place your left hand on your left shin.

3 Inhale and stretch your right arm upwards, palm forwards, keeping your hips stable and looking up. As you breathe here, open your chest more. Hold for several breaths, then slowly release.

Repeat on the other side.

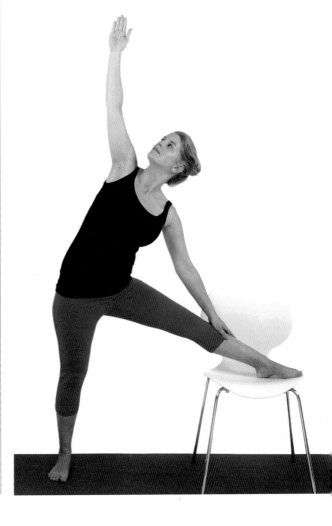

TREE POSE

Balancing postures such as Tree require strong alignment and create a sense of increased grounding, stability and centring. If your ankles and feet are feeling weak, use the supported version. If you are feeling strong, try the unsupported one.

1 Stand tall and strong, with your feet hip-width apart and parallel.

2 Inhale, lift your right foot and place the sole against your inner left thigh so that your right knee points outwards. Strengthen through your supporting leg and stretch your spine upwards.

3 Bring your hands to Prayer position in front of your heart, soften your eyes and look forwards. Hold the pose for several breaths.

4 If you are comfortable here, feel free to try alternate hand and arm positions such as arms raised above the head, whether in Prayer or shoulder-width apart, or arms directly out to the side. Hold your chosen position for several breaths and slowly release.

Repeat on the other side.

Variation: supported

1 Stand with a sturdy chair on your right. Rest your right knee on the chair and make sure the toes of your left foot are pointing forwards. Gently push your hips forwards so that your pelvis is tilted slightly under.

✳ **Tip**: As you gain hip, knee and ankle flexibility you will be able to place your foot higher up, towards the groin.

2 Inhale and stretch your spine up, keeping your neck long, and raise both hands to Prayer position in front of your heart. Hold for several breaths, feeling the sense of centring, then release.

Repeat on the other leg.

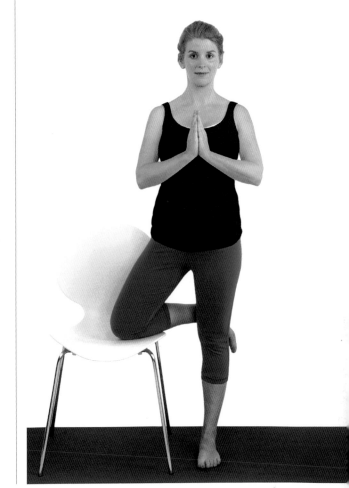

WIDE-LEG SQUAT

Squat poses create strength and stamina in the lower body. As such, they are fantastic preparation for labour: if the body feels strong, the mind can relax and let the birth process happen naturally. When performing squats, remember to breathe deeply and focus on the sense of centring and deep connection to your own body. Squats can be practised sitting on the edge of a chair or exercise ball, against a wall or freestanding but whatever level you are at, always maintain a firm grounding and make sure that major joints are aligned.

1 Sit on the edge of a chair or exercise ball with your legs wide, your feet flat on the floor and your toes pointing diagonally outwards. Alternatively, stand in a wide-legged stance and bend your legs as deeply as is comfortable, keeping your back straight and ensuring that your knees are over your heels and your feet point in the same direction as your knees.

2 Inhale and stretch both arms out and up above your head, then exhale and bring both arms slowly down until you touch the floor in front of you, placing one hand then the other on a thigh if needed for support during the transition. Repeat a few times moving slowly and steadily with your breath.

3 Then, with your spine upright, bring your hands into Prayer position slightly in front of your chest. Keep your shoulders down and elbows in line with your wrists. Firmly press your palms together and your feet into the floor. Hold for several breaths, feeling strong and centred, then relax.

Tip: Do not practise this sequence if you suffer from SPD or a low-lying placenta (see pp. 30–31).

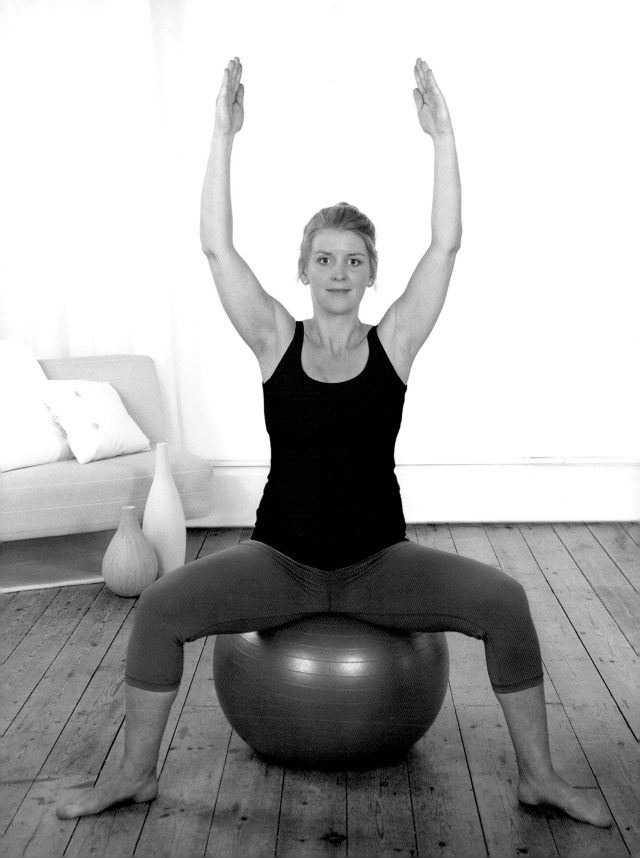

WIDE-LEG FORWARD BEND

Forward-bending helps to lengthen the spine, slow the heart rate, stimulate the sinuses and relax the mind. Physical balance can be affected during pregnancy, so if you are feeling unsteady, practise the supported version of this wide-legged forward bend, rather than the unsupported one.

1 Stand with your feet more than a metre (3 feet) apart and your hands on your hips. Inhale and raise both arms upwards, lengthening your spine.

2 Exhale, bring your hands down onto your thighs, bend your knees deeply, slowly lean forwards as your hips sink downwards, then aim to place your hands on the floor.

3 Gently walk your feet further apart until you feel a stretch between your legs. Inhale, straighten your legs and take more weight

into your hands. Bend your elbows if it feels comfortable and walk your hands forwards if you need more space. Keep pressing your feet down and feel your legs and spine stretch and open. Hold for several comfortable breaths.

4 With weight still on your hands, walk your feet inwards, bend your knees deeply, inhale and place one hand on your thigh, then the other, to bring your body slowly to an upright position.

Variation: supported

1 Position two chairs one in front of the other, facing the same direction about a metre (3 feet) apart. Sit on the edge of the back chair and open your legs wide. Ensure that your knees are over your heels and your toes are pointing in the same direction as your knees. Inhale and stretch your arms and spine upwards to create length and openness. Exhale and gently bring your arms down by your sides. Repeat several times.

2 Inhale, exhale and stretch your arms forwards, resting your hands, wrists or forearms on the top of the other chair. Keep stretching through your spine and arms and be sure not to let your chest collapse. Hold for several deep breaths, then relax.

3 Exhale, gently lower your hands, arms and head towards the floor, placing your palms down if possible and bending your elbows if you have space for your abdomen. Rest here for several breaths, then release slowly.

Tip: If suffering from low blood pressure, be sure to release out of the posture very slowly on an inhalation.

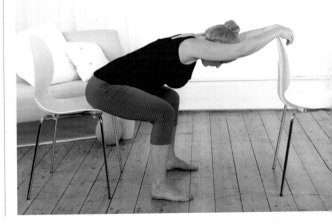

ARM AND LEG EXTENSION

The Arm and Leg Extension is a great way to enhance your balance at the same time as getting a lovely stretch from a safe, stable, kneeling position. There is also plenty of room for your baby bump when you are on all fours.

Tip: Remember, if ever you need a rest between postures, go into Child's pose (see p. 122) and relax for a few deep breaths.

1 Come into a tabletop position, on all fours, with your knees directly under your hips and your wrists under your shoulders, palms down and fingers spread out, index fingers pointing forwards.

2 Walk your knees together slightly. Exhale and lift your right leg straight behind you, then inhale and extend your left arm in front of you, so that your arm, spine and leg are all on the same level. Look straight down, keeping your head in line with your arms. Hold for several breaths.

3 Inhale and raise your left arm up by your ear, lower your right leg down to the floor behind you, with toes touching the ground, and stretch from your foot to your hand. Exhale and release back to tabletop position.

Repeat on the other side. Practise two or more cycles.

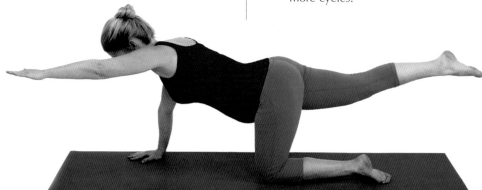

BOW

As your bump grows, more pressure will be placed on the front of your body. This posture allows you to create maximum opening through the front of your body to counteract the physical effects of this. However, it involves both strength and balance, so should only be practised if you feel entirely stable and comfortable with it.

1 Come into a tabletop position, on all fours, knees directly under your hips and wrists under your shoulders, palms down, fingers spread out, index fingers pointing forwards.

2 Walk your knees together slightly. Fix your gaze slightly ahead of you on the floor. Exhale and lift your right leg straight behind you to hip level and hold for several breaths.

3 Bend your right knee and bring your heel in towards your head.

4 Press your right hand firmly into the floor, inhale, lift your left arm and reach backwards to take hold of your right foot.

5 On your next inhalation, feel your front side expand as you gently push your right foot up and away from you, keeping both shoulders pointing forwards. Hold for several breaths, then release slowly.

Repeat on the other side. Practise two or more cycles.

Tip: If the final stages of this pose feel too strong, just do it to step 3, hold for several breaths, release and repeat on the other side.

GENTLE PLANK

Gentle Plank helps to build awareness of proper alignment of the spine and pelvis. It also tones your forearms, shoulders and chest, as well as gently strengthening your abdominal muscles, so is good for conditioning the belly in pregnancy, as well as helpful for regaining muscle tone after birth.

Tip: If you have SPD, practise Gentle Plank with your knees and thighs together and think about keeping all your energy aligned through your centre.

1 Come into tabletop position, on all fours, knees directly under your hips, toes tucked under, and your hands slightly in front of your shoulders, palms flat and fingers spread out, index fingers pointing forwards. Straighten your arms, but try not to lock the elbows, and keep your spine long.

2 Inhale, gently pull your stomach muscles in and tilt your pelvis under, then bring your bodyweight forwards so that your shoulders come directly over your wrists. Ensure that you move your shoulders away from your ears to open your chest. Drop your hips down so that your spine becomes straight and look forwards to keep your neck in line with your spine.

3 Hold for several breaths, then exhale and return to tabletop position. Repeat several times if you feel strong, building up repetition as you get stronger. Finish by resting in Child's pose (see p. 122).

EASY PUSH-UP

Many women focus solely on strengthening the lower body in preparation for labour. However, it is also vital to strengthen the upper body – not only so that the torso can expand to accommodate the growing baby and the chest can stay open for easy breathing, but also so that you feel fit and strong enough to cradle and support your newborn baby after birth. Easy Push-up will help you to develop this strength.

1 Slowly come into Gentle Plank position (see opposite), focusing on good alignment.

2 Then exhale and bend your elbows back lower your upper body down until your chest is at elbow height.

3 Inhale, push firmly into your palms and bring your body back up.

Repeat five times for one set and then rest in Child's pose. Over time, build up to three or four sets resting in between each one.

Tip: If this is too hard, it's fine to let your elbows come away from your body slightly as you lower down. But as you gain more strength, try to keep your elbows moving in and back.

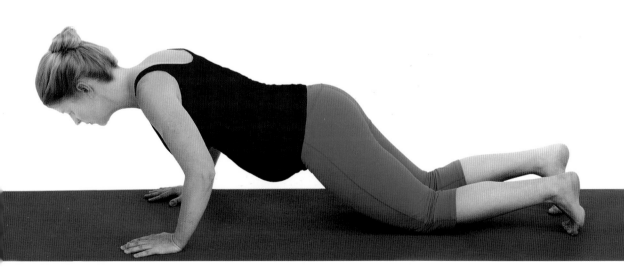

PIGEON POSE

Pigeon pose is a kneeling stretch that allows for a slow, deep expansion of the pelvic, hip, buttock and lower back muscles. It should be practised in a relaxed way to allow you to notice the subtle opening of your birthing muscles. It is also recommended for sciatica (see p. 31).

1 Gently come into tabletop position, on all fours, with your knees directly under your hips and your wrists under your shoulders, arms straight, palms flat and fingers spread out, index fingers pointing forwards. Your spine should feel long.

2 Inhale and carefully bring your left knee forwards so that it rests on the floor behind your left wrist and your heel is in front of your right hip.

3 Exhale and slowly slide your right leg back along the floor until you feel a stretch in your hips. If your hips feel stiff, keep your weight through both hands, and make sure that your hips remain at equal height.

4 Inhale and lift your chest up slightly to increase the sense of opening in your front body as well as to tone your back muscles.

5 Exhale, then inhale and raise your left arm upwards, feeling a stretch from your fingers to your toes. Hold for several comfortable breaths, then release.

Repeat on the other side.

Tip: Use a cushion or block under your extended front thigh and hip for support and comfort if hips are lifted up off the floor.

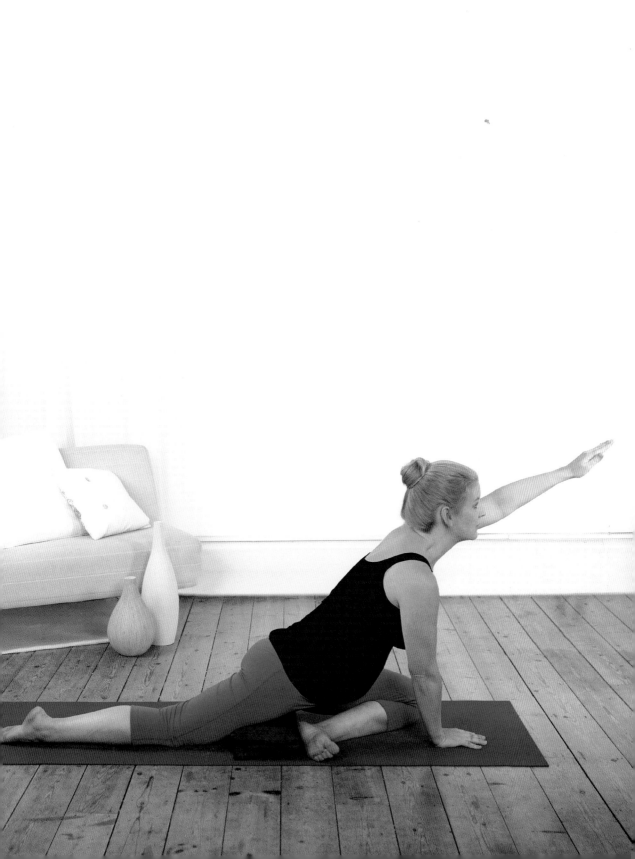

RECLINING
TWIST 1

This twist is a great way to release pressure from your back, neck and shoulders and to balance out your spine. Twisting will also refresh the central nervous system which helps to relieve fatigue. It is important that twisting postures focus on the upper back so as not to compress the stomach area.

1 Lie down on your back with cushions or pillows behind your head (and upper back if needed), and also on either side of your thighs for comfort.

2 Keeping your legs together, bend your knees, place your feet flat on the floor and bring your arms out to the sides at shoulder-level, palms and shoulders down, to stabilise your body.

3 Inhale, then exhale and slowly lower your knees towards the right. You can place your right hand under your right knee to gently guide your knees down if desired.

4 Once in position, bring your right arm out to the side again and gently turn your head towards the left. Hold for several breaths, then release slowly using your arm for support if needed.

Repeat on the other side. Practise the posture a couple more times if you feel comfortable.

RECLINING TWIST II

This one-leg twist is a progression from the double leg version and allows you to fully experience opening your body from its core. As you lie in this position, take time to appreciate the cleansing and balancing effects of spinal twists.

1 Lie down on your back with cushions or pillows behind your head (and upper back if needed), and also on either side of your thighs for comfort.

2 Keeping your legs straight and feet apart, bring your arms out to the sides at shoulder-level, palms and shoulders down, to stabilise your body.

3 Exhale, then inhale, bend and raise your left leg up, placing your foot onto the floor on the outside of your right knee.

4 Exhale and slowly lower your left knee over the cushion on the right, turning your head to the left. Hold for several breaths, trying to maintain a straight line from your head down through your outstretched leg.

5 Inhale and slowly lift your left knee up and release the leg.

Repeat the twist on the opposite side. Practise this cycle two more times.

✳ **Tip**: Relax back to your starting position after this posture but bring your feet together and let your knees open to a Butterfly position (see p. 46).

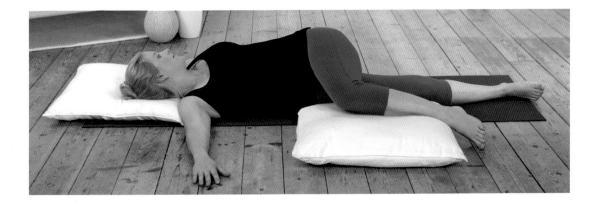

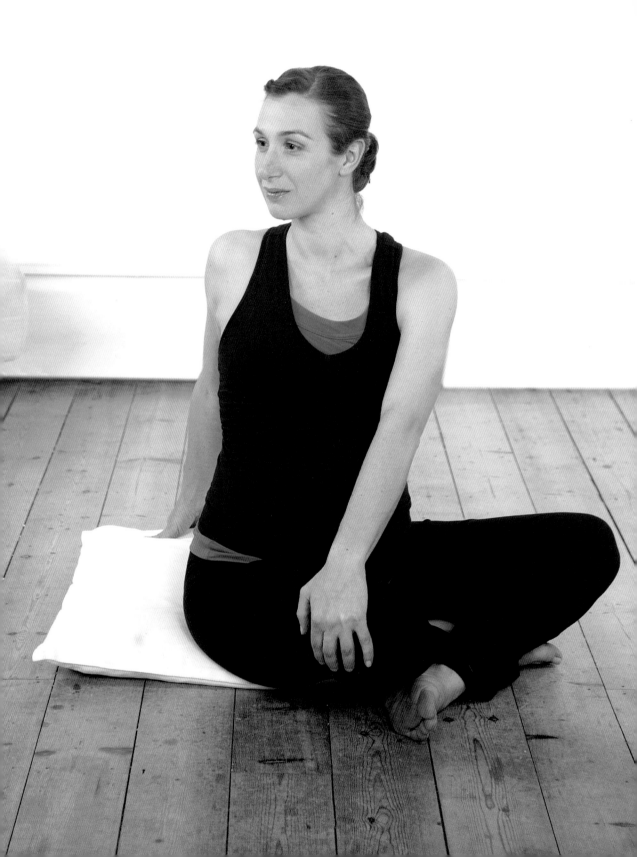

THIRD TRIMESTER POSTURES

This final stage of your pregnancy is when your baby is fully maturing, in readiness for arrival into the outside world. As he or she is reaching full weight, your job is to stay comfortable, relaxed and both physically and mentally fit. Your yoga practice should therefore now be about maintaining strength and flexibility, staying balanced and focused, and preparing yourself mentally for the birthing process.

You can practise the following postures at any time during your third trimester to help with this, choosing the most appropriate variation of each to suit your ever-changing needs. Just always remember to start with the Sun Salutation sequence to warm up and end with the Relaxation sequence to unwind.

Practising the breathing, meditation and visualisation techniques on pages 130–139, to complement the postures in the following pages will help you to remain calm, open-minded and enjoy the final journey towards the arrival of your precious gift.

KNEELING FORWARD STRETCH

This kneeling forward stretch creates a lovely sense of length in the spine from a nice stable base. The wide-knee position gives more room for the increased size of your bump, as well as a greater opening for your hips.

1 Gently come into a tabletop position, on all fours, but open your knees slightly wider than hip-width apart and bring your toes to touch each other.

2 Exhale, bend your elbows so that you lean on your forearms and turn your right hand inward to make a right-angle at your elbow.

3 On the next exhalation, stretch your left arm forwards until your left palm and your forehead rest on the mat with your bent right arm above your head.

4 On the next exhalation, stretch your shoulders back away from your ears and gently push your tailbone back and up. Hold for several breaths.

Repeat on the other side.

KNEELING LION

Sitting on your heels in this posture will help to stretch the tops of your feet, ankles, shins and across the knees – areas that can get stiff from extra baby weight and that can also suffer from water retention in the third trimester. Performing the facial stretch will relieve pressure in your face, neck and shoulders, which will feel so good, you won't want to stop.

1 From a tabletop position, bring your knees wide and your toes to touch each other, exhale and gently sit your hips back onto your heels. Place your palms or fingertips on the mat in front of your knees so your arms are straight.

2 Inhale and lift your head and chest up, opening your front side and keeping your elbows soft and shoulders down.

3 Exhale, stick out your tongue, look upwards and 'roar' like a lion with a deep 'ahhh'.

4 Inhale and drop your eyes and head. Repeat your lion face a couple of times or more if it feels good.

Tip: This pose is excellent for releasing tension in the face, throat and neck and also fear from the mind.

DEEP SQUAT
IN PRAYER

In the later stages of pregnancy as the body becomes more flexible through hormonal changes and weight becomes greater, creating stability in your practice becomes more important. Practising this deep squat, which brings you closer to the floor, will keep your centre of gravity lower for more solidity. The position is also excellent for encouraging your baby into the birthing position, but do not practise it if you have SPD or a low-lying placenta.

1 Begin in a tabletop position, on all fours, with your toes tucked under. Walk your hands back towards your knees and gently start to lift your knees up. Your hips will drop down and your weight should shift over your heels, so that your feet become flat on the floor. Keep your toes turned slightly outwards in line with your knees.

2 Inhale and lift one hand and then the other, bringing your palms together in Prayer position (*anjali mudra*, see p. 39) in front of your chest. The back of your arms should be against the inside of your knees creating resistance between these two points. Look forwards and keep your spine straight. Inhale and feel your spine lengthening and chest lifting, exhale and feel your feet grounding down and your hips and pelvis opening. Hold the pose for several breaths, then reverse out of it.

Tip: Practise against a wall if needed for support and place a folded towel or yoga blocks under your heels if they don't rest comfortably on the floor.

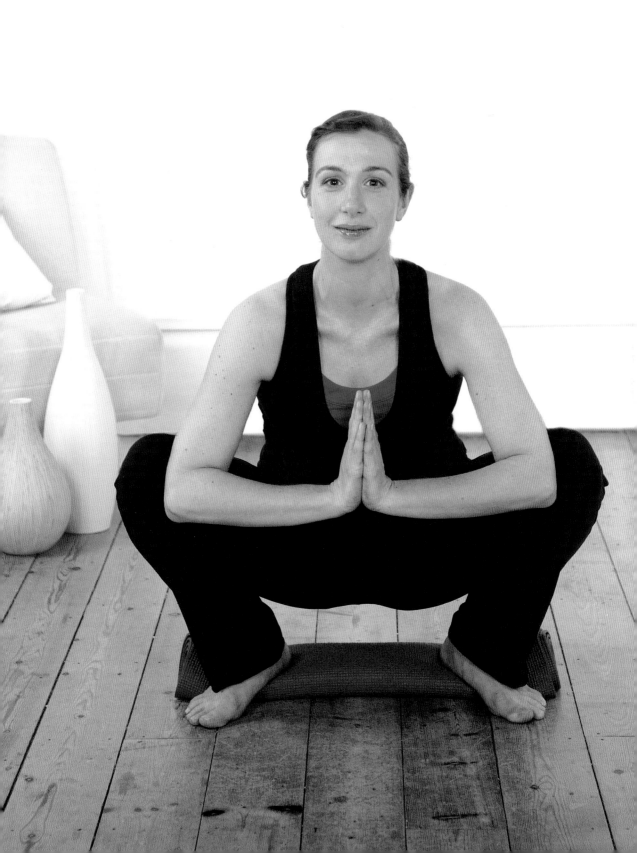

STANDING HIP ROLLS

Hip-rolling postures are ideal preparation for labour. The rocking and rolling action that they involve will encourage greater mobility of your hips and pelvis as well as enhancing blood flow to these areas and to your baby. Hip rolls can also be used during labour gently to release pressure on the back.

1 Stand in a wide-legged stance facing a wall, with about 60–80cm (2–3ft) between you and the wall.

2 Place your hands flat on the wall above shoulder height, spread out your fingers and push the wall.

3 Exhale and rock your hips back so your arms are extended. Bend one knee and then the other to roll your hips in a clockwise motion, working with your breath. Repeat several times in one direction, then switch to doing it counter-clockwise.

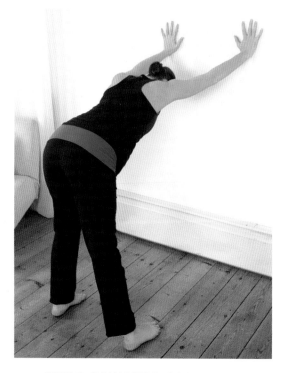
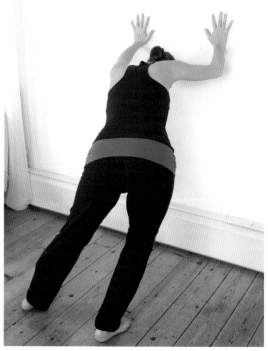

Variation: sitting hip rolls

1 Sit on an exercise ball or the edge of a sturdy chair, with your feet wide apart and flat on the floor, toes pointing diagonally outwards. Place your palms on your thighs with fingers pointing outwards.

2 Exhale and begin gently rolling your hips in a clockwise direction so that the soothing rhythm matches your breathing. Then reverse and do it in the other direction. Repeat for as long as feels comfortable.

Tip: Remember to keep your shoulders down and your chest open and lifted.

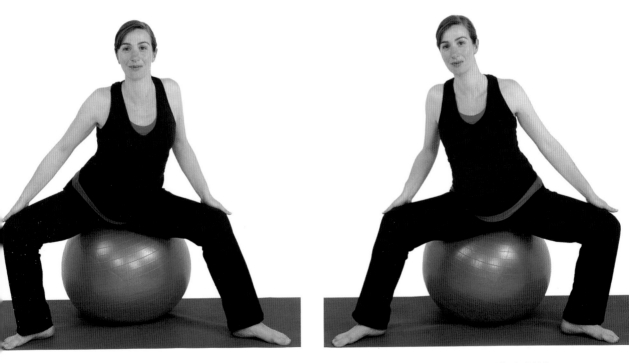

SINGLE-LEG SEATED STRETCH

Seated stretches help to encourage flexibility of your pelvis and hips in preparation for the birthing experience, as well as releasing any tension in your lower back and groin areas, which is common in the later stages of pregnancy.

1 Sit sideways on your mat, place your palms behind you on the floor and extend your right leg out. Raise your bent left knee in the air, place the foot flat on the floor, and place your left hand around your left knee. There should be a wide opening between your legs.

2 Inhale, sit up and flex your right toes back. Then exhale and reach your right hand down to hook your big toe with your two index fingers. If you can't reach, use a belt or strap.

3 Inhale and lift your pelvic muscles, then exhale, relax them and release the toe and knee grip.

4 Lower your left knee onto the mat and bring your heel in towards your groin. With hands on hips, inhale, sit up, keep your shoulders back and down, then exhale and reach for your big toe with your right two index fingers. Again, if you can't reach, use a belt or strap.

Tip: If it is difficult to keep your chest open and shoulders down in step 5, place the upward reaching arm behind your back and try to grab the opposite thigh with your hand, in a bound arm position. Inhale and open the shoulders and chest more.

5 Exhale and bend your right elbow down towards the floor. Inhale and raise your left arm directly upwards, palm facing forwards, until you feel a stretch on your left side. Hold for a few breaths, then slowly release.

Repeat the whole sequence on the opposite side.

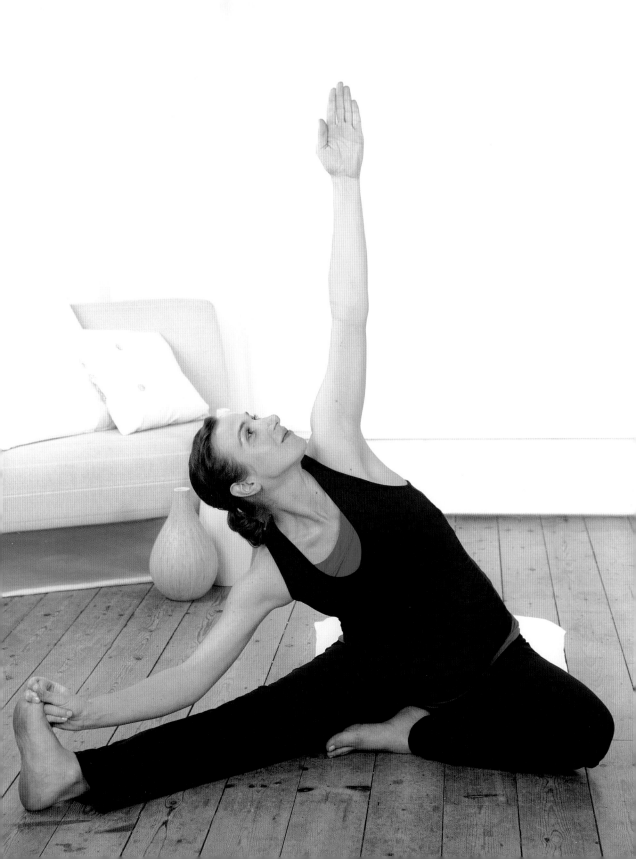

PULLING THE ROPE

The deep side stretch that this movement offers creates a sense of space throughout your chest and sides, conditioning your middle back and toning your abdominal muscles. Having your legs open wide not only gives you a strong, stable base from which to work but also creates a stretch in your hamstrings and hips, which are important to keep strong and flexible in preparation for labour.

1 Sit in a wide-leg position on your mat with your palms behind you on the floor. Tilt your pelvis slightly backwards and sit up.

2 Inhale and reach up with your right hand, exhale and gently bring the arm down the midline of your body, slightly in front of you, as if pulling a rope. As you reach the bottom of the rope with your right hand, reach up to start pulling it with your left hand.

3 Continue these flowing arms movements as if you were pulling or climbing a rope until you feel you have had a good stretch.

CHURNING THE MILL

This movement involves a circling action that helps to further tone your back and abdominal muscles and encourages increased blood flow to your hips and pelvis, as well as building greater flexibility in these areas.

1 Sit in a wide-leg position on your mat with your palms behind you on the floor. Tilt your pelvis slightly backwards and sit up.

2 Inhale and bring both hands together at waist-height in front of you with your fingers and thumbs interlaced, and begin to move your hands in a clockwise motion in front of you as if stirring a cauldron: first move your arms and body to the left, then forwards, then to the right, and back. Repeat several times, then reverse the direction.

Tip: If these poses feel too strong with both legs open, try them with one leg bent instead but make sure you maintain balance by switching legs and doing the same number of movements on each side.

STRETCH WITH WALL SUPPORT

By now your yoga practice will have loosened your pelvis and hips to prepare you for this stronger, wide-leg stretch, which is invaluable in the run-up to the birth to ensure both optimal strength and flexibility. It is important here to practise a high level of awareness in order not to overstretch.

1   Sit with your back against a wall, on a low cushion or blanket for comfort if desired. Place your hands on the backs of your thighs and gently open your legs wide so that your knees are bent and feet flat on the floor.

2   Place your hands on the floor by your hips for support. Inhale and stretch your spine, chest and head up. Exhale and gently open your knees wider, pressing your hips down and back a little until you feel a stretch in your inner thighs.

3   Hold for several comfortable breaths, gently pressing your shoulders back into the wall and letting your knees open more on each exhalation. Then use your hands under the thighs to release your legs slowly.

Repeat once more.

STRETCH FACING THE WALL

When you feel ready for a deeper stretch still, this wide-legged posture facing the wall is ideal. Be sure to begin slowly and with awareness. Then, as your legs and hips soften, gently move your hips forward for a deeper opening. Remember never to push too hard. With practice, this stretch is slow, long, deep and feels amazing.

1 Sit down cross-legged facing a wall. Place your hands on the floor behind you and gently open your legs wide and straight. Slowly move your hips forwards until the soles of your feet meet the wall and you feel a stretch in your inner thighs.

2 Inhale, stretch your spine, chest and head up. Exhale and gently lean forwards to feel the stretch. Inhale again and lean forwards more. If you want to increase the stretch, cross your arms on the wall and rest your head on your arms. Hold for several breaths or longer at your deepest stretch, then use your hands to release your legs slowly and reverse out.

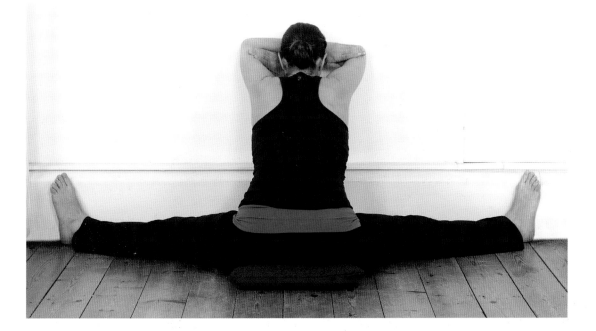

CROSS-LEGGED TWIST

Doing spinal twists in your final few months of pregnancy will help to maintain a flexible spine, which will counteract the pressure that carrying extra weight places on this area. As the spinal column is opened, energy will move more freely through your body, giving you the necessary fuel to deal with fatigue and physical stress.

1 Sit cross-legged on your mat. Place your left hand on your right knee, inhale and stretch your spine, chest and the crown of your head upwards. Exhale and twist to your right bringing the fingertips of your right hand to rest on the floor behind your back.

2 Inhale and stretch up, exhale and twist. Hold the final twist for several comfortable breaths, and reverse out.

Repeat on the other side.

Tip: If you want more of a stretch, reach your right hand around your back to hold the opposite inner thigh, in a bound arm position.

Variation: zig-zag twist

This zig-zag leg variation of a spinal twist gives you all the benefits of the cross-legged twist, but at the same time provides a valuable stretch across your knees, thighs, hips and also through the sides of your body.

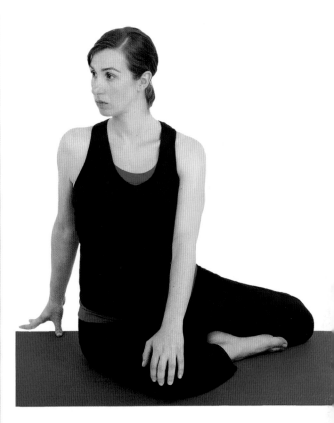

1 Sit on your mat with your knees bent to the right and your feet positioned to the left, so that your right sole rests against your left thigh.

2 Place your right hand behind you on the floor and your left hand on your right knee.

3 Inhale and lift your chest and body upwards. Exhale and twist to the right. This twist is not as deep for the spine but you will feel it more over the hip and torso.

4 Inhale and stretch up again. Exhale and twist slightly further. Hold for several comfortable breaths, then release.

Repeat on the other side.

 Tip: If two knees bent to the side is difficult, keep one leg straight and the other bent.

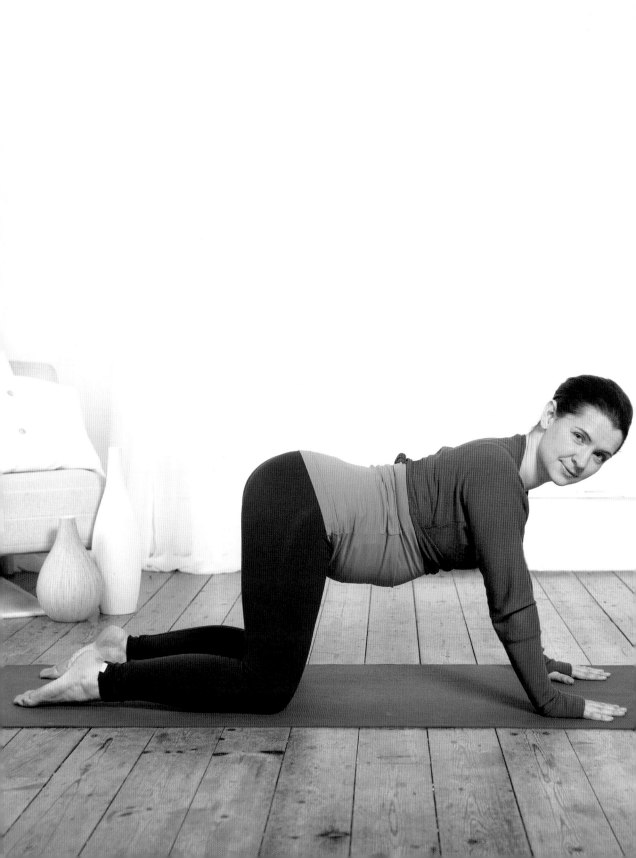

POSTNATAL POSTURES

Following the big birth, life is completely transformed with the beauty of your new child, the physical strain from the birth and the changes and challenges that lie ahead.

The first six weeks is a time to focus on deepening the bond between you and your newborn by continuing to practise breathing and relaxation techniques with your baby lying on or near you. As your body is still reacting to the birthing process remember to think about proper alignment of the spine when sitting or standing and keeping the pelvis stable by moving slowly and evenly.

As your body starts to recover more in the 6–12 week postnatal phase, you can begin to resume a gentle yoga practice using the specially chosen postures in the pages that follow, depending on how you feel. Gradually build up strength over time, starting with the first few postures and the Gentle Flow sequence (see pp. 104–107). Do not push it, especially if you have had a C-section or any complications during birth, as your body needs time to heal properly, which can take several months. As your natural energy and vitality return, you can begin to practise the Standing Flow sequence (see pp. 108–111) and beyond, as well as incorporating some of the more gentle postures from your prenatal practice. Be sure to finish any session with the relaxation poses recommended.

NECK ROLLS

During the first few weeks after giving birth, your body can feel rather unbalanced, and the new challenges of breastfeeding and carrying your baby are likely to place pressure on your neck, shoulders and back. Neck Rolls will help to release this tension, which will, in turn, help to balance the skeletal, muscular, endocrine and nervous systems.

1 Sit up straight on a chair or cushion on the floor. Keep your shoulders down and chest open. Inhale and gently roll your head to the right and then slightly backwards. Exhale and continue to roll your head to the left and forwards.

2 Repeat this circular movement several times, then reverse the neck rolls in the opposite direction.

Tip: If you want to do this exercise when your baby's with you, hold him or her with both arms as you do it.

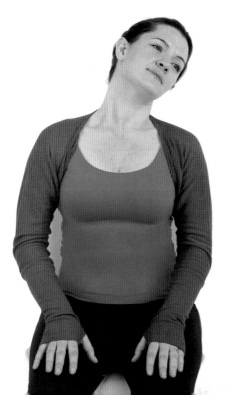
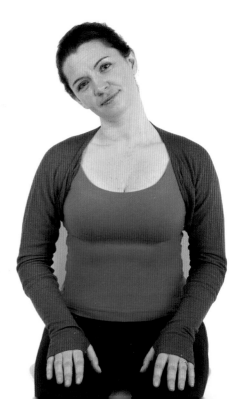

SHOULDER ROLLS

These gentle Shoulder Rolls will help to create a further sense of opening in the upper body and counteract any feelings of stiffness, heaviness and tension in the head, neck and shoulders. Remember to start slowly and build up the amount of repetitions as you become more aware of where the maximum tension is.

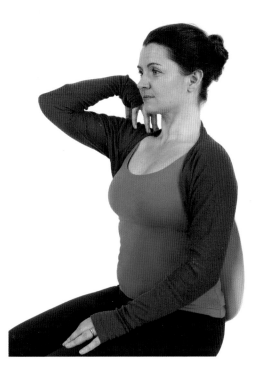

1　Sit up straight on a chair or cushion on the floor. Inhale and roll your right shoulder forwards, then up towards your ear. Exhale and slowly roll the shoulder back and down. Repeat this circular shoulder motion several times.

2　Bend your right arm so your fingers rest on the top of your right shoulder. Inhale and circle your elbow forward and up. Exhale and circle the arm back and down. Repeat this circular motion several times.

Repeat both movements on the other side.

✳ **Tip**: If you want to do this exercise when your baby's with you, hold him or her first in your left arm, then in your right.

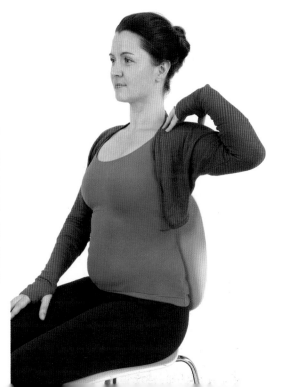

GENTLE FLOW SEQUENCE

This gentle but dynamic sequence of postures provides a great re-entry into your yoga practice after the birth of your baby. Remember to begin slowly, breathe deeply and move with your breath. Proper breathing will give you energy, focus and internal conditioning that will support you as you rebuild your strength. Aim to practise the sequence daily once you feel ready, building up the amount of times you flow through the poses as you become stronger.

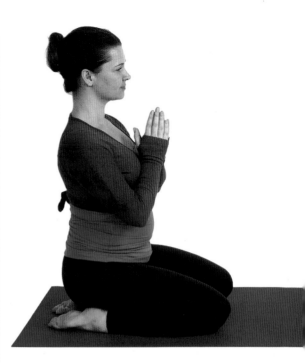

Kneeling prayer

1   Begin by sitting on your heels with your hands in Prayer position in front of your chest.

2   Inhale and raise your arms upwards. Exhale and stretch your arms out to the sides, then down towards the floor.

Child's pose

3 Inhale, place your hands on the floor in front of you and gently come into a tabletop position, on all fours.

4 Exhale and sink your hips back to your heels into Child's pose (see p. 122). After birth, knees can be closer together as your bump gets smaller.

Mini chaturanga

5 Inhale and move your body weight forwards over your hands. Exhale and bend your arms, allowing your chest to drop close to the floor. Inhale, lift your chest up and rock your weight back until you are in tabletop position again.

Tip: If you are at home alone with your baby, place him or her in a safe position near you as you practise so that you can make eye contact or reach him easily if he starts to cry.

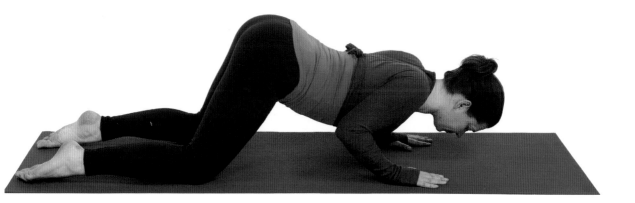

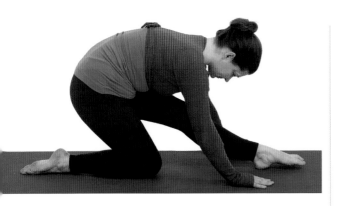

Kneeling stretch

6 Inhale, pull in your stomach muscles and step your left foot forward between your hands. Keep your hips in line, both facing forward, and your left knee directly over your left foot.

7 Exhale, straighten your left leg, press your toes towards the floor, sink your hips back and extend your arms forwards. Gently bring your head and upper body forwards and down towards your front leg until you feel a stretch on your hamstrings, hips and back.

Kneeling warrior

8 Inhale and shift your body weight forwards, so that your knee is bent and properly aligned over your left foot. Tuck your right toes under.

9 Keeping your hips stable, slowly inhale, raise your body up and stretch your arms upwards. Look straight ahead and, as you breathe, create more length in your spine. Hold for several breaths.

✳ **Tip**: Keep hands resting on the front thigh if raising the arms feels too difficult at the beginning stage.

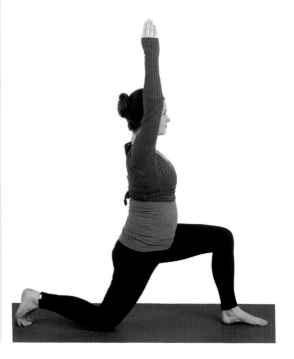

Child's pose

10   Exhale, slowly bring your hands down to the
floor, gently step your left leg back and rest
in Child's pose (see p. 122) for a minute.

Repeat steps 6–9 using the opposite leg.

Tip: Remember to rest in Child's pose at any time
during the sequence if you feel fatigued. It is
important to remember not to push yourself.

STANDING FLOW SEQUENCE

With regular practice the Gentle Flow sequence will help you to regain your strength and stamina. When you feel ready to attempt a more vigorous set of postures, try the Standing Flow sequence in the following pages, remembering to focus on alignment and stability as your body still needs to be treated with care as it rejuvenates after the birth.

Mountain pose

1 Stand in Mountain pose (see p. 34), with your hands in Prayer position, and close your eyes. As you breathe become aware of your alignment, your feet grounding into the floor and your spine stretching up.

2 Inhale and raise your arms over your head.

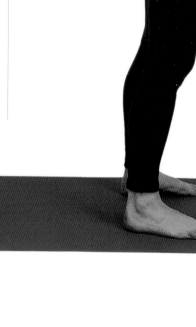

Forward bend

3 Exhale and fold forward with your knees slightly bent. Place your hands on the floor, shoulder-width wide, close to your feet.

Downward dog

4 Inhale and pull in your stomach muscles. Exhale and step your right leg back and then your left leg to Downward Dog (see p. 36). Hold the pose for several comfortable breaths.

5 Still in Downward Dog, gently bend one knee and then the other several times as if you were bicycling your legs. Then exhale and press both heels down towards the floor again, stretching your feet, calves and legs for several more breaths.

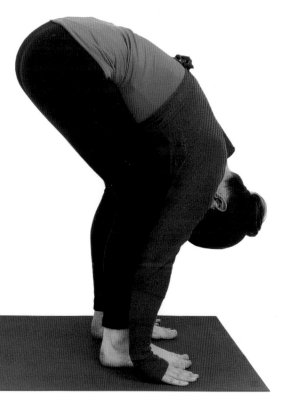

Mini chaturanga

6 Bend your knees and gently come down to kneel on the floor in tabletop position, on all fours. Exhale, bend your arms and allow your chest to lower close to the floor. Inhale, lift your chest up and rock your weight back until you are in tabletop position again.

7 Exhale and sink your hips back to your heels into Child's pose (see p. 122) and rest for several breaths.

Downward dog

8 Raise your body, tuck your toes under, firmly press your palms into the floor and as you exhale raise your hips into Downward Dog.

Tip: Keep your knees bent in Downward Dog if the pose feels too intense. Focus more on lengthening the spine first and then stretching the legs.

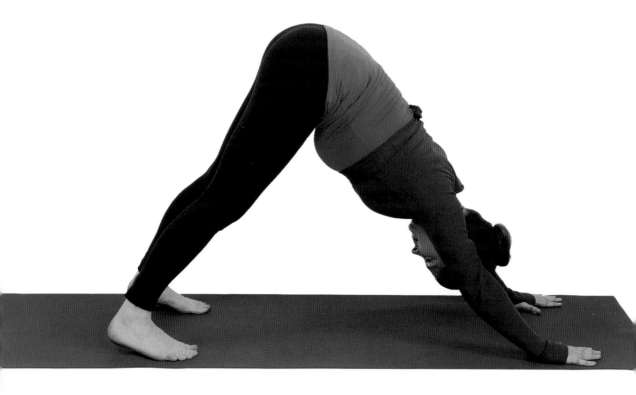

Deep squat

9 Slowly walk your feet in towards your hands, keeping your feet hip-width apart or more. Exhale and slowly bend your knees so that your hips lower into Deep Squat in Prayer (see p. 88). Hold for several comfortable breaths.

10 Place your hands on the floor, and keeping your knees bent, slowly raise yourself up to standing.

Mountain pose

11 Inhale and raise your arms above your head. Exhale and bring your arms down.

12 Finish in Mountain pose, with hands in Prayer position and breathe deeply.

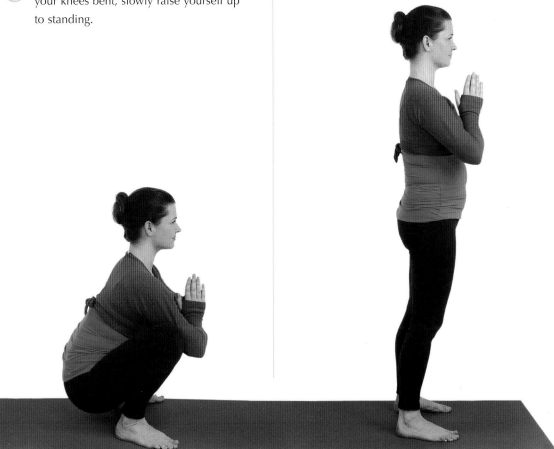

GENTLE TWIST

Gentle twisting poses will start to realign your spine and tone your waist and lower back muscles after birth. They will also help to stimulate the central nervous system, which can help with low energy levels as a result of lack of sleep and physical strain.

1 Sit up straight on a chair with your feet flat on the floor, or on blocks, and knees and feet together or open, whichever feels more comfortable. Inhale and stretch your spine up from your lower back through to the crown of your head and gently pull in your stomach muscles.

2 Exhale and twist your torso, upper back and head to the right and place your right arm or hand on the back of the chair, keeping your left hand on your knee or thigh.

3 Inhale and stretch up further through your spine, exhale and twist deeper. Hold at the maximum twist for several breaths, then release.

Repeat on the other side.

Tip: If you want to practise this pose when your baby's with you, hold him or her on your lap, first with your left arm, then your right.

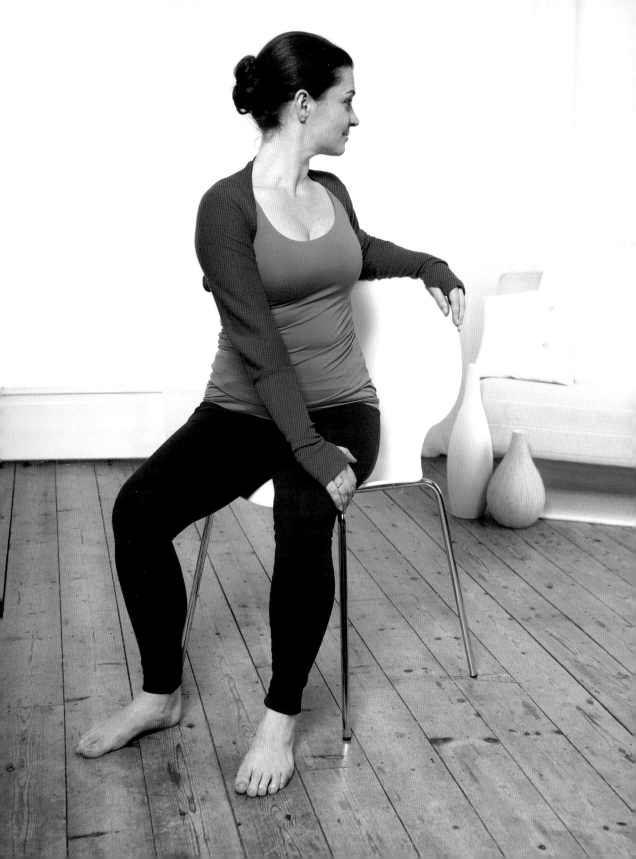

CAT AND DOG TILT

These postures will help to condition your pelvic and abdominal muscles after birth, allowing you to restore core stability as quickly as you can. Use slow, deep breathing to move consciously between the positions and focus on accessing all areas of the spine.

1 Gently come into a tabletop position, on all fours, with knees directly under your hips and wrists under shoulders, palms flat and fingers spread out, index fingers pointing forwards. Your spine should feel long.

2 Inhale and ensure your shoulders are down, then exhale and tilt your pelvis under while dropping your head down with your chin tucked in. This will create an arch in your back like an angry cat, hence the name Cat Tilt (see below left).

3 Inhale, then exhale and gently tilt the pelvis back, lift your head up and return your spine to a neutral position. Inhale and lift your eyes and head further up, tilting your hips further back and allowing your spine to curve slightly downward into Dog Tilt (see below right). Keep your stomach muscles engaged, hold for a moment, then release. Repeat the Cat and Dog Tilts several times.

4 From the Dog Tilt, exhale and move both your head and upper body to the right and your hips towards your head until you feel a stretch through your left side and a gentle compression through your right side. Hold for several breaths. Inhale and release to the centre. Then repeat on the opposite side. Practise these side stretches several times and keep building up repetitions as your stomach muscles become more conditioned.

Tip: Cat and Dog Tilts are also good positions in which to practise Kegel exercises – important internal muscle movements that help to restore pelvic control after birth.

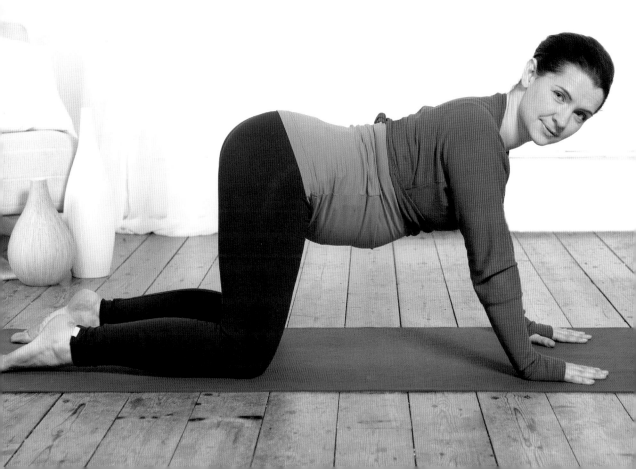

GENTLE SIDE PLANK

Slow and steady movements that support the body are best when you are reconditioning your body after birth: when the body is stable, the muscles can be activated correctly, and strength will return more efficiently. Postures that might have felt easy before pregnancy will probably feel very difficult so a pose like Gentle Side Plank is ideal as it will help to rebuild core muscles.

1 Lie on your right side with your legs and feet stacked on top of each other (knees can bend a little if it feels more comfortable). Rest your weight on your right forearm, with your left arm and hand extended forward and palm facing down on the floor in front of you.

2 Inhale, suck your stomach in and raise your weight off the right shoulder so you feel it extend. Exhale and slowly lower your shoulder back down. Repeat several times.

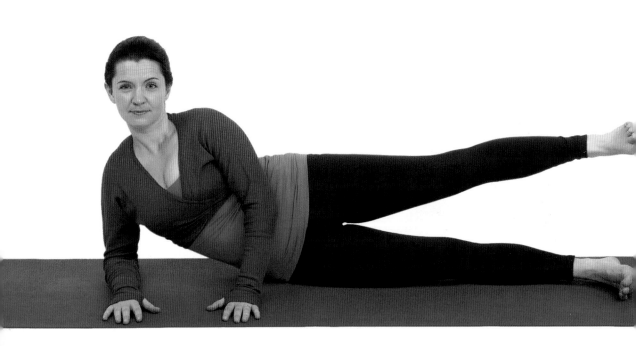

3 Straighten your left leg, flex your left foot, inhale and slowly raise your leg up while keeping your hips stable. Exhale and lower your leg. Repeat 3–4 times.

4 Straighten your right leg on the floor, bend your left knee and cross it over the right leg so that your left foot is flat on the floor. Inhale and press your right forearm and feet firmly into the floor, extend your right shoulder and gently raise your hips off the ground to a supported side plank position.

5 Hold for a breath and gently release. Repeat one more time.

Repeat the whole sequence on the other side.

Tip: Remember that you can always stop at step 3 if the final stage is too challenging at first.

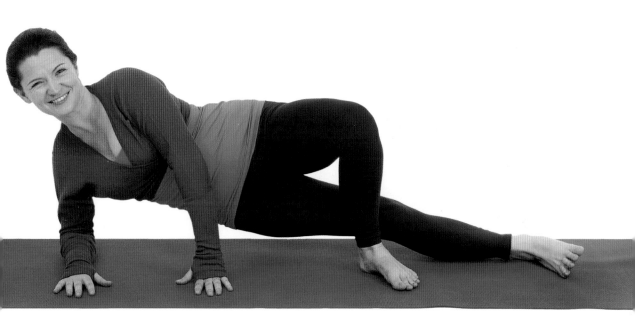

SEATED STRETCHES

The following poses allow you to remain in a secure, stable position as you focus on good alignment, the lengthening of muscles and creating more of a sense of space in your body. Your body will still feel fairly flexible because relaxin remains in the body for approximately five months following the birth, so be sure to practise these stretches with heightened awareness.

1 Sit upright on the floor and extend your legs straight in front of you.

2 Inhale and stretch your arms upwards as you pull in your stomach muscles. Exhale and stretch gently forwards towards your toes. Repeat several times and hold the stretch at its deepest point for several comfortable breaths.

Tip: When rebuilding back and tummy strength, for some it might be difficult to stretch forward with raised arms, so walk your hands along the legs to your deepest stretch. You can also use a strap around the feet.

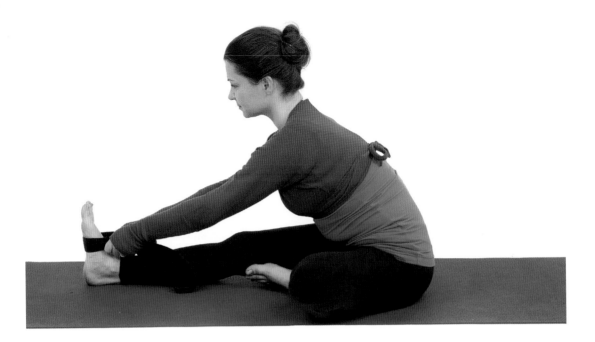

3 Loop a strap or towel around your right foot and bend your left knee out to the side so that its sole is against your right inner thigh. Inhale and stretch your spine upwards as you pull in your stomach muscles. Flex your feet, exhale and gently lean forward leading with your chest and hold for a few comfortable breaths. Repeat the stretch to go deeper and hold at your strongest level. Repeat on the opposite leg.

✳ **Tip**: As your natural flexibility returns, you will be able to walk your hands closer to your feet in step 3 until one day you can omit the strap in step 3.

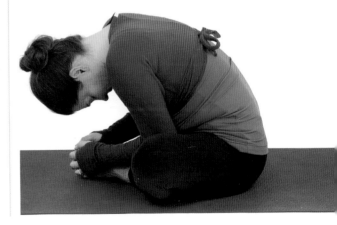

4 Bring both legs to Butterfly (see p. 46) with the soles of your feet touching. Place your hands behind you on the floor. Inhale and stretch your spine up and engage your core muscles. Hold your feet with your hands, exhale and gently lean forwards over your legs. Relax your head down and breathe in this seated forward bend. Hold for several breaths, then release slowly.

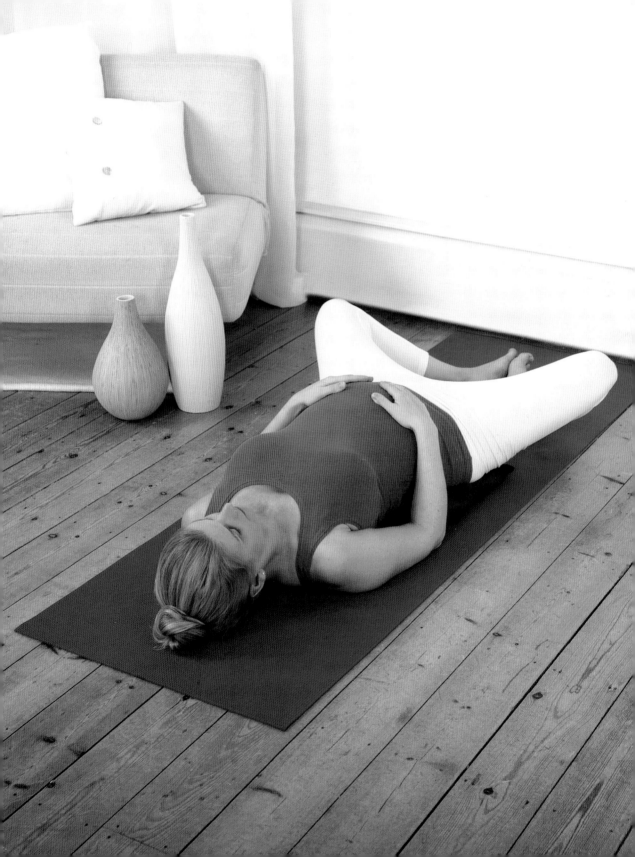

RELAXATION POSTURES

Stress is the body's natural response to the many demands placed on it. During pregnancy, when both the body and the mind have to deal with many dramatic changes, levels of stress often increase. As high levels of stress can cause health problems, learning to consciously relax and let go of this stress is invaluable as it will help to keep you calm and balanced, supporting the healthy growth and birth of your baby.

The relaxation poses in the pages that follow are a key component of any yoga session, as rest is just as important as physical activity for a well-rounded practice. In fact, it is while practising relaxation poses that the work you have done in the physical postures and breathing exercises will really take effect on both the body and mind.

Be sure to do Corpse pose (see p. 128) at the end of every yoga session but also feel free to practise the other relaxation poses any time you feel tired, stressed, imbalanced or a little overwhelmed by everything. Towards the later stages of pregnancy, relaxation methods are particularly useful as they will enhance and preserve your energy in preparation for the birth and impending motherhood.

CHILD'S POSE

This forward-bending relaxation posture creates a sense of nurturing, calm and restoration for both body and mind, which makes it perfect to practise at any point before, during or after a yoga session, on its own during a stressful period of the day or at any point during your pregnancy or postnatal period. It allows you to fully relax your front body, which in pregnancy is heavily stressed, while extending the back side of your body. Placing your head below your heart in this pose also gives your heart a chance to rest, lessening any strain on the cardiac system.

1 Gently come to a tabletop position, on all fours. Bring your big toes to touch keeping your feet flat and toes extended. Your knees should remain open to accommodate your baby bump.

2 Exhale and gently sink your hips back to rest on your heels. Extend your arms fully forward, with palms flat on the floor, and gently rest your forehead on the mat. If you want to take on an even more restful position, place your arms down by your sides and turn your palms to face upwards.

3 Breathe deeply in this position for as long as you need to.

4 To release, inhale, press your palms into the floor and lift your head, body and hips back to tabletop position. Open your feet and either push into Downward Dog (see p. 36) on an exhale or sit your hips down to your heels and raise your chest and body up.

Tip: If you feel any discomfort in your ankles, place a folded towel underneath the front of them for support.

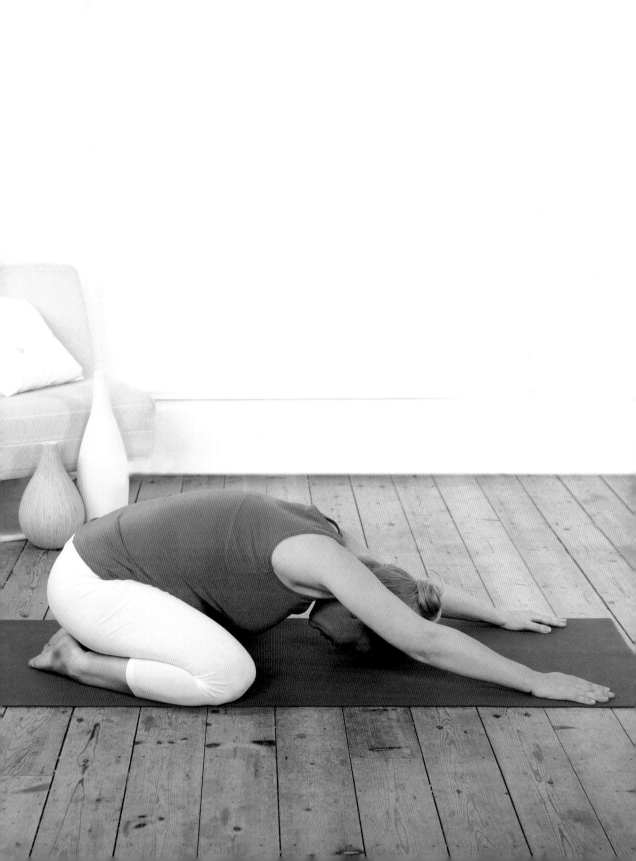

LEGS UP THE WALL

This is a passive posture that benefits the body by allowing your legs to relax and the blood to flow backwards to relieve pressure on your veins, muscles and joints. The position is also beneficial for swollen feet, varicose veins, Restless Leg Syndrome (see p. 31) and mild backache. It is best practised up until you are around 30 weeks pregnant when it is still comfortable to lie on your back.

1 Place a low cushion or folded blanket on the floor close to a wall. Gently bring yourself to lie on your back with your hips resting on the cushion about 15–20cm (6–8in) away from the wall.

2 Rest your legs up the wall with a 30–60cm (1–2ft) gap between your feet. Your legs should be close to a 90-degree angle with the floor, and your hips, back and head fully relaxed.

3 Inhale and stretch your arms above your head on the floor, as you gently stretch your legs by flexing your feet. Relax your feet, hold the stretch and breathe deeply for about five seconds.

4 As you breathe, rock your pelvis from side to side several times to relax your hips and back. Stop in a neutral hip position and bring your arms down by your side.

5 If you would like to repeat, slowly release into Side-lying Corpse (see p. 129), rest, then try again. To release properly, roll onto your left side with your knees bent, then slowly come onto all fours to transition to another movement.

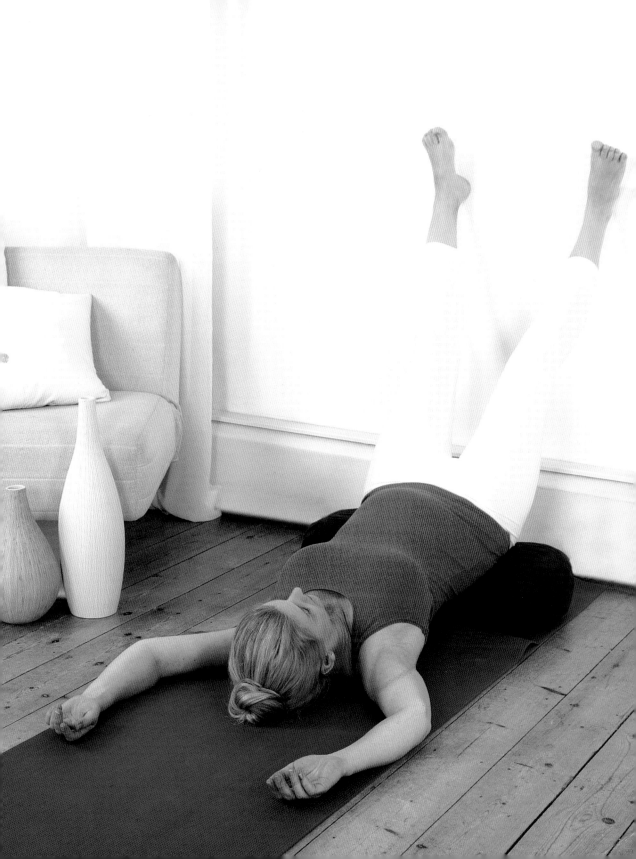

LEGS UP THE WALL IN BUTTERFLY

As your baby develops and its weight increases spending time relaxing on your back should be limited, so best to come out of Legs Up the Wall for a few minutes, rest in a foetal position lying on your left side and then progress to Legs Up the Wall in Butterfly position. These postures can be practised in sequence, or independently.

1 Place a low cushion or folded blanket on the floor close to a wall. Gently lie on your back with your hips resting on the cushion about 15–20cm (6–8in) away from the wall.

2 Rest your legs up the wall with a 30–60cm (1–2ft) gap between your feet. Your legs should about 90-degrees to the floor, and your hips, back and head fully relaxed.

3 Exhale and bend your legs so that your knees point outwards and the soles of your feet come together in a wide Butterfly position. Rest your hands on your stomach. Relax more deeply here on every exhale. Hold for one to two minutes maximum.

4 To release, roll onto your left side with your knees bent, then slowly come onto all fours to transition to another movement.

SUPINE BUTTERFLY

Supported relaxation poses let you release tension, nurture yourself and develop an openness that will help you throughout your pregnancy. Even practised for just a few precious moments, postures such as Supine Butterfly will restore and revitalise you for the daily challenges of pregnancy and impending motherhood.

Tip: Place cushions under your knees for added support if you need it, and/or fold two blankets lengthwise and fold back the top end as cushioning for your neck, shoulders and back.

1 Place a low cushion or folded blanket on your mat. Gently bring yourself to lie on your back with your middle back resting on the cushion and bend your legs, with your feet flat on floor.

2 Bring the soles of your feet together and let your knees open as wide as feels comfortable. Gently rest your hands wherever feels comfortable.

3 Close your eyes, mentally scan your body for tension and release it with the next exhalation. Stay in this position for a maximum of two minutes, then gently open your eyes and release slowly.

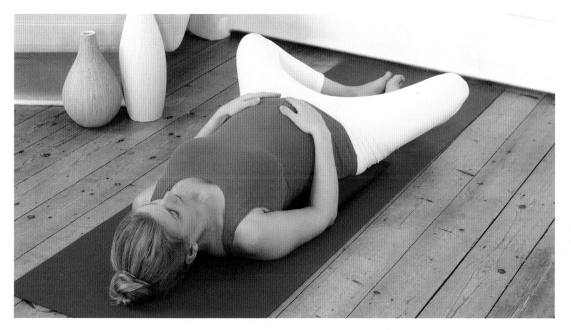

CORPSE POSE

Corpse pose, also known as *Savasana*, is the classic yoga relaxation position. Practising this posture is essential to get the most out of your yoga practice as it allows time for both your body and mind to recharge. Try to spend at least 5 to 20 minutes a session in this relaxation pose while you are pregnant to nurture both yourself and your baby. Traditional Corpse pose, on your back, can be practised until about 30 weeks, but then it's best to practise Side-lying Corpse to relieve pressure on the vena cava – the main blood vessel that carries blood back into the heart.

1 Lie on your back and place cushions or bolsters under your knees and head to allow your spine to align properly and get comfortable. Let your knees open gently outwards.

2 Place your hands softly over your pelvis and join your thumb and index fingers to make a triangle.

3 On every exhalation, relax your body. On every inhalation, welcome in positive thoughts, energy and vitality. Continue this for as long as feels comfortable, then open your eyes and slowly come out of the posture.

Tip: Remember that on days when you have less energy, a yoga session can simply be a combination of breathing and relaxation exercises. Keep it simple but consistent.

Variation: side-lying corpse

1 Slowly lie down on your left side, resting both your head and right knee on a cushion or pillow (the pillow for your right knee should be just in front of your left leg). If needed place another cushion between your arms for comfort.

2 Allow your body to fully relax as you close your eyes. On every inhalation, welcome in energy and positivity. On every exhalation, release tension, stress and negative thoughts.

3 Allow yourself to physically and mentally relax here for a few minutes. Then open your eyes and slowly come out of the posture.

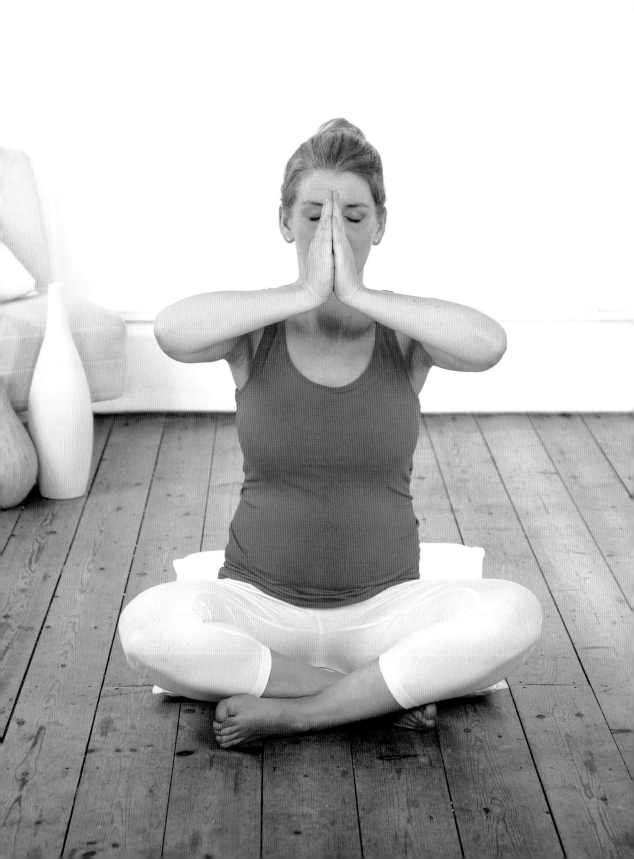

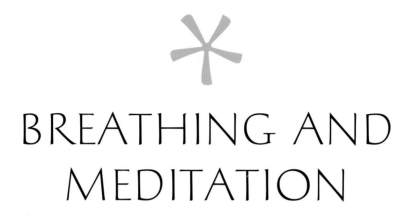

BREATHING AND MEDITATION

A mother-to-be not only has to acknowledge the physical changes occurring in her body but also the mental and emotional shifts as she perhaps starts to worry about the birth and what impending motherhood will be like.

One of the main benefits of practising yoga during your pregnancy is developing an understanding of the connection between the mind and body. If the body is under stress, breathing usually becomes quick and the mind starts racing. Conversely, if breathing is strained and the mind is under stress, such as when a mother feels fearful about labour, the body will tighten up, making the experience harder. It's therefore just as important to work on the mind as it is on the body to achieve a state of positivity and equilibrium.

The yogic breathing and meditation techniques in the pages that follow will allow you to do just this – calming your mind, helping you to keep your emotions in balance and encouraging an open attitude to change. Simply practise the exercises any time you feel the need, though remember that you should not practise full breath retention during pregnancy, so only hold the breath briefly and exhale fully.

SUN BREATH

Sun breathing is a stimulating breath that helps to increase
energy and vitality. This exercise is therefore helpful to boost
energy levels, to create a sense of warmth in the body, to
alleviate feelings of anxiety and to make the mind more alert.

Sit in a comfortable, upright position. Close your eyes if it feels right and
breathe naturally.

Rest your right hand on your right knee, keeping your hand relaxed and open,
whether face up or down.

Raise your left hand and place your thumb gently against your left nostril.
Breathe in slowly, taking a full breath through your right nostril.

Gently close your right nostril with the ring finger of your left hand. Hold for a
second, then slowly release the ring finger and breathe out through your right
nostril until your lungs are empty.

This is one round of breathing. As a beginner, practise 10 rounds. As the
breathing technique becomes more comfortable, increase the duration
to 3–5 minutes.

MOON BREATH

Moon breathing is a cooling breath – the opposite to Sun breathing. This exercise is useful to cool and calm the body and mind, and is especially useful during pregnancy when heightened hormone activity and increased blood supply can increase body temperature.

Sit in a comfortable, upright position. Close your eyes if it feels right and breathe naturally.

Rest your left hand on your left knee, keeping your hand relaxed and open, whether face up or down.

Raise your right hand and place your thumb gently against your right nostril. Breathe in slowly, taking a full breath through your left nostril.

Gently close your left nostril with the ring finger of your right hand. Hold for a second, then slowly release the ring finger and breathe out through your left nostril until your lungs are empty.

As with the Sun Breath, start with 10 rounds and increase duration with experience.

BLOWING A FEATHER BREATH

This is a gentle cooling breathing technique that can be practised at any time you feel heavy, hot and bothered. Practising it will help to slow down your heart rate and not only cool you down but also relax both your body and mind. It is particularly useful during labour, too, when physical exertion creates a great deal of body heat.

Sit in a comfortable upright position and bring one hand close to your mouth, with the thumb and index fingers together, as if holding the end of a feather. Purse your lips and inhale slowly through your mouth. Then blow out gently, making a soft 'hoo' sound, as if blowing the imaginary feather. Your fingertips should feel a cool breeze.

Repeat until you feel calmer and cooler.

CANDLE BREATH

Just before the second stage of pushing begins during labour, it can be useful to slow the natural urge to push too soon, and this technique can really help with this so practising it throughout your pregnancy is great preparation for the big day.

Sit in a comfortable upright position and raise one hand towards your face, picturing each finger as a candle.

Imagine that your body feels an urge to push your baby out too soon. Then hold off this urge by exhaling in short puffs or blows in order to extinguish the five candle flames, one at a time. Repeat as necessary.

THE GOLDEN THREAD BREATH

This breathing technique involves using a visualisation to promote a sense of calm in both the body and mind. Invaluable any time you feel a little stressed or overwhelmed, it is also particularly useful during labour as focusing on the exhalation is key to pain management.

Sit in a comfortable upright position and breathe naturally, inhaling through your nose and exhaling through slightly parted lips.

As you exhale, imagine you are slowly and carefully blowing a fine golden thread out of your mouth, relaxing deeply as you do so. As you inhale, breathe in oxygen and vital energy for you and your baby.

As you exhale, imagine the breath – and thread – gradually getting longer, moving further away from you, until it can reach no further. Then once again gently breathe in. Experience the breath flowing in and out, creating a sense of healing energy.

BIRTHING VISUALISATION

Practising this visualisation throughout your pregnancy will help to create a positive mindset about the birthing experience, which will help you to deal with the strong physical impact when the day comes. Encouraging you to focus on the joy of meeting your new child, it is most useful in the third trimester and also during labour itself.

Lie down in a comfortable position using pillows and bolsters for support if desired. Place your hands gently on your stomach, close your eyes and focus on your natural breathing.

Start to visualise the onset of labour, with contractions happening slowly. Imagine that each contraction is a wave on the ocean. As you inhale, the wave starts to crest and rise to its highest point as the contraction gets stronger. As you exhale and the contraction starts to susbside, you ride the wave gracefully towards your baby, who is waiting on the shore to meet you. Each wave – although strong and powerful – is taking you closer to meeting your child.

At the end of the visualisation, imagine sitting on the beach with your baby cradled safely in your arms, opening its eyes and smiling at you.

Then gently open your eyes and relax.

BUTTERFLY MEDITATION

This liberating meditation can be practised at any time during or after pregnancy when you feel in need of a sense of comfort, support and vitality. It is best practised when you are tired so that you can fully relax and enjoy the feeling of being nurtured and re-energised.

Lie down on your left side, using pillows and bolsters to make yourself comfortable if desired. Wrap a blanket around yourself so you don't feel cold.

Settle into a rhythm of slow and steady breathing. As you do so, visualise a small caterpillar slowly crawling up a tree, resting on a vibrant green leaf and, over time, spinning a cocoon around itself made of golden, silken thread. When the caterpillar is fully covered, focus deeply on the cocoon.

Breathing more deeply, now visualise yourself inside the cocoon. Feel the warmth, security and stillness of this safe, enclosed space. Remain here as long as you need to, until you sense a transformation happening with each deeper breath: an energy growing inside you, making you feel stronger and lighter.

As this energy increases you cannot be contained by the cocoon. See it start to break open and feel the light and radiance surrounding you. You are a beautiful butterfly that can fly or float anywhere you choose.

When you feel ready, slowly open your eyes, take a deep breath and stretch before slowly sitting upright.

WELCOMING
THE BABY MEDITATION

This meditation will help to make a deep mental connection between you and your baby. The hand position (or *mudra*) involved is called *anjali mudra*, or Prayer position. *Anjali* means 'offering', so you are giving an offering to your unborn child for it to enter your life. You may wish to do this exercise with your partner.

Sit in a comfortable upright position and press your palms together in front of your nose. Elbows should point straight out and be parallel to the floor and the tops of your middle fingers should be in line with your eyebrows.

Close your eyes and focus on the spot between your eyebrows (the Third Eye).

As you inhale fully, welcome your baby with openness and compassion. As you exhale, release any tension or negative thoughts. Make each inhalation deeper and feel your baby becoming happier and more secure within your family.

Continue this for several minutes. When finished, gently lower your arms and stretch your body.

ABUNDANCE MEDITATION

This meditation will cultivate a sense of openness and gratitude about both your own health and that of your baby. It can be practised at any time during your pregnancy, labour or after the baby is born and is especially useful if you are experiencing any feelings of negativity.

Sit in a comfortable, upright position, such as cross-legged on the floor or kneeling with your spine straight.

Cup your hands so that your little fingers touch each other and bring your hands about 15cm (6in) in front of your heart centre. Gently lower your gaze with a soft focus on your palms.

As you slowly and deeply inhale, visualise your palms becoming full of positive energy, abundance and health. As you exhale, just relax. Each inhalation will make the hands become fuller, until they are overflowing.

Practise for several minutes, and end with a deep inhalation, then a full exhalation.

RESOURCES

When practising yoga during pregnancy, there are a number of resources you may find useful and supportive, from finding your nearest classes to where to buy yoga equipment, as well as books and websites that offer more information about helping you stay healthy throughout your pregnancy.

Equipment

Yoga Matters
32 Clarendon Road
London
N8 0DJ
Tel: 020 8888 8588
www.yogamatters.com

The Yoga Shop
25 Rodney Street
Edinburgh
EH7 4EL
Tel: 0870 066 4202
shop.theyogashop.co.uk

Yoga-Mad
Units 2-4 Willersey Industrial Estate
Willersey
Worcestershire
WR12 7RR, UK
Tel: +44 1386 859550
www.yogamad.com

Asquith London
7 Leamington Road Villas
London
W11 1HS
Tel: 020 7792 9414
www.asquithlondon.com

Books and references

Chopra, Deepak *Perfect Health* (Bantam, 2001)
Gaskin, Ina Mae, *Ina Mae's Guide to Childbirth* (Vermilion, 2008)
Iyengar, B.K.S *Yoga the Path to Holistic Health* (Dorling Kindersley, 2007)
Motha, Dr. Gowri and Swan MacLeod, Karen *The Gentle Birth Method*, (Thorsons, 2004)
Murkoff, Heidi E. and Mazel, Sharon *What to Expect When You're Expecting* (Simon & Schuster, 2009)
Romm, Aviva *The Natural Pregnancy Book: Herbs, Nutrition and Other Holistic Choices* (Celestial Arts, 2003)
Saraswati, Swami Satyananda *Asana, Pranayama, Mudra, Bandha* (Bihar School of Yoga, 1969)
Strom, Max *A Life Worth Breathing* (Skyhorse, 2010)

Websites

www.homebirth.org.uk
www.babycentre.co.uk
www.birthlight.com
www.holisticlocal.co.uk
Junomagazine.com
www.localyogaclasses.co.uk
www.nhs.uk
Wombecology.com

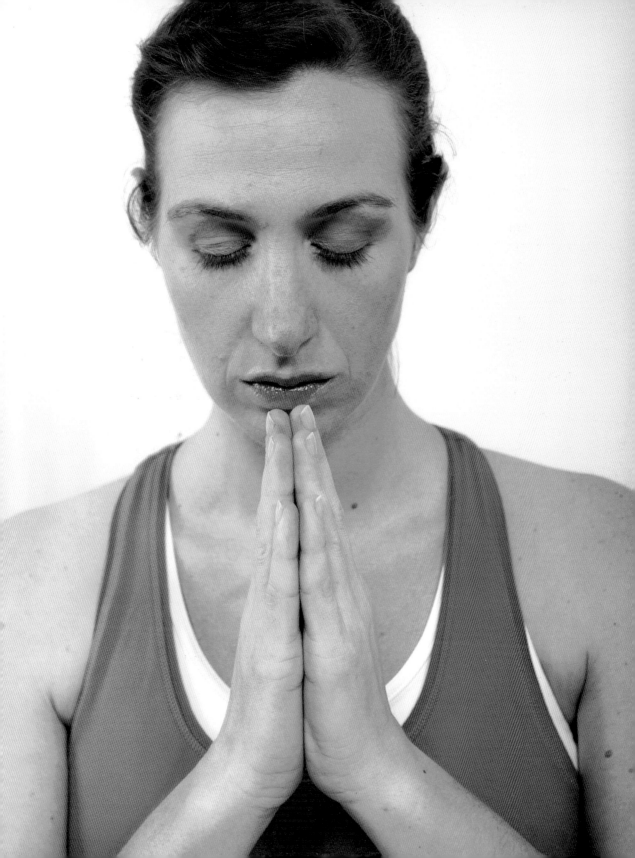

INDEX